For Such a Time as This

Alysia Rieg

WESTBOW
PRESS®
A DIVISION OF THOMAS NELSON
& ZONDERVAN

WestBow Press books may be ordered through booksellers or by contacting:

WestBow Press
A Division of Thomas Nelson & Zondervan
1663 Liberty Drive
Bloomington, IN 47403
www.westbowpress.com
1 (866) 928-1240

ISBN: 978-1-5127-2919-1 (sc)
ISBN: 978-1-5127-2920-7 (e)

Library of Congress Control Number: 2016901725

Print information available on the last page.

WestBow Press rev. date: 3/22/2016

Contents

This book is dedicated to
The One who inspired it, God, the I AM. It is because of
God that I have been transformed. It is only because of my
Lord and Savior that I have stepped into my destiny. May
this book be not only for YOUR glory and honor but may
it also exalt your name. Thank You for choosing me.

To my family and friends who supported
me, encouraged me, loved me.

To my enemies and even to those whom I cared so dearly
for who God has allowed to cross my path to abandoned
me, to reject me, to discount me, to not have chosen me. I
thank God especially for you because had you not mistreated
me, God would not have set a table before me and I may
have never been able to help others become overcomers.

For Such A Time As This

Esther 4:14

Grieving over the loss of a loved one is one of the most traumatic experiences any one person can go through. To lose someone you love very much, who holds a valuable place in your life, who in your heart and mind are irreplaceable; is one of many things in life that can bring you to a place where you are not only alone, but find yourself feeling scared, broken, empty, lost, hurt, discouraged, angry, uncertain, and left with a mind filled with so many unanswered questions.

Loss can come in many forms: neglect, abandonment, death, or divorce, to list a few. No matter the vehicle used to lose the person you love, it all comes with the same emotions, feelings, thoughts, and your heart as well as your world is left shattered, into a million little pieces. Not to mention, the time it takes to heal feels as if it is everlasting.

My biggest and most painful loss, came by way of a divorce, after an almost nineteen year marriage. Though loss of any kind is extremely painful, being somewhat partial, I would share that, in my opinion and experience, divorce is the most painful of all the different forms of loss. I think being left by choice hurts deeper than when someone leaves you unintentionally.

Having suffered a severe devastating loss, I understand whole-heartedly how you feel and what you are going through.

Empathetically, I know the pain of your heart just as intimately. Your mind, like mine was, is permeated with many unanswered questions. Questions that begin with the word why; "Why is this happening? Why did they leave me? Why did they lie? Why didn't they keep their word? Why do they think someone else is better than me? Why won't they fight for our relationship? Why is he/she so selfish? Etc." Your questions then turn inward, causing you to question your own worth: "Why am I not worthy of their love? Why am I not good enough or even enough? Etc." These questions will then cause your mind to lead your feelings and then you begin to "feel." You feel like you failed, like a failure. You feel ashamed or embarrassed. You feel unworthy or that you have no worth. You don't feel attractive, maybe even ugly. You feel unloved, possibly even unlovable. These feelings of "less than" will bring you to a place of inadequacy: your self-esteem begins to fall or becomes non-existent, you may no longer like yourself or how you look. You will become angry, scared, hurt, lost, hopeless, insecure, and you will be all of these, all at the same time.

On top of these thoughts and feelings you are struggling through, you may have some people in your life who are telling you to "Cheer up, pick yourself up, you deserve better, it's his or her loss, this happens to everyone so get over it, if God wanted you to be together you would be," etc. Then there are the others who may abet you to gossip about the person who didn't choose you and elicit the sharing of your situation, many will solicit unwanted opinions and advice, telling you what they think you should and or shouldn't do. You will also have "friends" who choose the other side and who will leave you, "friends" who will talk about you and your business to anyone and everyone, maybe even "friends" who will "pray" for you and your situation with others. Then, you will have those friends who will choose your side and if you, by chance, are fortunate enough to have true friends, friends who will be there to support you, encourage you, and pray with you, friends who genuinely have your best interest at heart who will also, in love, tell you when you are wrong, count yourself blessed.

Through all of this you will hurt and you will be sad, you will be misunderstood, you will be angry, maybe even destructive, you will be confused, and more than likely you will want to be the victim, you will feel alone, you may even feel suicidal and you will get tired of people telling you what they think, how you should feel or what you should do. You will want to be justified and you will want your revenge.

Trust me, I know your pain all too well. I was there, right where you are right now and I am here to tell you as a living testimony, that there IS a God who loves YOU, who adores you, who treasures you, who finds you precious and worthy enough to fight for, enough to die for.... and He did!

As I shared a few paragraphs ago, I was married almost nineteen years to the love of my life, the father of my three beautiful children. He walked away from me for some female. In my assured opinion, she wasn't better than me in any way, but for some reason she was "better" enough for him to walk away from me, from all of his promises, from our family, from our children for whatever she had to "offer." I was left broken, empty, lost, devastated, confused, scared, angry, full of hate and vengeance. I contemplated death but knew I still had responsibilities as a mother of three children, children who didn't ask for any of this and who definitely did not deserve to come from a broken family. I had no one who was choosing me, who would fight for me, yet I knew I had to fight, doing it with no hope, no plan, and no strength for three people who needed someone to fight for them. But I couldn't do it. BUT GOD! God whispered to me, He picked me up, He cleaned me up, He fought for me, He redeemed me, He told me who I was and whose I was. He loved me. He chose me and He gave me the strength that I needed to fight for three innocent people, who deserved to be fought for.

This program that I have designed will take you through the measures that God led me through that brought me to healing and peace, to a heart that is once again alive, to a life that is worth living, and more importantly, a testimony that surpasses extraordinary. I will be as transparent with you as I can be and I will share with you in raw form exactly, what I went through mentally, emotionally, and physically and how God used all of it to help me go from broken to blessed for His glory. I am going to remind you of who you are and whose you are. You will see and know that you are worthy, valuable and special. By the end of this program, you will know without a shadow of a doubt why you were created and what your life means, you will be an overcomer; an empowered and victorious conqueror and you will be ready to really begin living your life to it's fullest, desiring to fulfill the purpose for which you were created; a champion that finishes the race that was laid before you, if you follow this program exactly.

Throughout this book, I will teach you what is true (I will bold it for you, feel free to highlight them with a highlighter as you go) so that you can better know, enabling yourself to be equipped to battle these moments of extreme sadness, brokenness, and hopelessness.

One thing you must understand before you can continue reading on is, this too shall come to pass. You are NOT alone and what you are going through is NOT who you are, it does NOT define who you are or whose you are, nor does it define who you will become or where you will go or what you will do with your life.

Your history does not define your destiny.

Also know, that there is no such thing as a coincidence. You are reading this at the exact appointed time that you need to be reading it; you are reading it because it is **FOR SUCH A TIME AS THIS.**

Dear Reader,

*Whether you are a Christian or not, I ask that you make the effort to read my entire book without allowing your beliefs or unbeliefs to get in the way of the words I write to you. I ask that you please finish the entire book and then draw your opinions or decisions. My words are not to try to convert you into becoming a Christian, though I am a Christian. The words I have written in this book are simply the affairs of my heart. Though the names of the people have been changed, I write to you with complete honesty and the thoughts and feelings that I share are raw and real. The story I share with you is not a religious one, it is the truth, this, my reader, is MY testimony, the redemptive story of **my** life. ALL of us have a story, so I humbly ask that you read on with an open mind and a receptive heart. I want to sincerely say in advance, thank you for taking the time to read my most inner thoughts and for walking through the pains and the joys that I have endured. I thank you for taking the time to step into my life and becoming a part of this leg of my journey. I pray that all that I have had to endure; the loss and grief, the endless pain and hurt, each trial I went through, every test I had to take, all of the betrayals that left wounds in my back and in my heart, and my complete devastation and loss brings you healing or at least gives you hope, or maybe becomes the light at the end of your dark tunnel. Know this one true fact: I survived, I am a survivor, I came out victorious, a strong overcomer and you, my, friend can too! May God's will be done in your life as it is being fulfilled in mine. Many blessings.*

Much love,

Alysia xoxo

Chapter 1

REJECTION

*"If the world hates you, know that it
hated me before it hated you."*
John 15:18 (NIV)

The dictionary defines rejection as (1.) the act or process of rejecting (2.) the state of being rejected. (3.) something that is rejected. The dictionary does not do a very good job of defining what rejection truly is. Rejection is an extremely painful sentiment that cuts intensely and runs extremely deep. Rejection takes much time to heal from and many never heal from it. When you're heart has been stabbed with the sharp point of rejection it tends to have an extremely difficult time clotting and continues to bleed unremittingly, even when bandages are applied in attempt to hold the lacerated pieces of your tattered heart together, the pain of rejection always seems to find a way to seep out of the frayed edges.

I felt the razor sharp edges of the blade of rejection when it sliced open my heart, dismembering it into many pieces, over and over. To have someone you love, throw you by the wayside is not only devastating, but also, tormenting and excruciatingly painful; not just to your heart, but to your mind, and even to your soul.

As I have already shared, my husband leaving me was the most devastating and the most destructive thing that has ever happened to me. Thinking back to that Saturday in August, I can remember vividly the instance his words were put into action, making it my reality. We had just flown back from a trip on the east coast having had a nice flight and drive home from the airport. As soon as we walked in the front door, he grabbed a few things and then turned to our three children and to me and told us he was leaving. He said, "I need to be happy." He was leaving us for a female (throughout the book I will refer to her as female and not as a woman because a real woman would not and does not take part in destroying a family and certainly walks away when the wife tells her to leave her husband and her family alone) whom I will call "Ema." Then he literally turned his back on us and walked out of the door.

I remember standing there frozen, trying to get his words to process in my mind. I quickly remembered that my children were standing behind me, so I turned around to look at my children only to witness my two daughters in tears and anger on my son's face. Rejection had immediately sliced their hearts the minute their father's words came out of his mouth. My teenage son angrily demanded, "Mom, let's just leave and move to Texas." My son knew from his years of growing up with me that family was number one only after God and his first instinct in that moment was to run home to family. I answered him, "We don't run from our problems, we face them and we work through them." Looking back now, I sometimes wonder if I had made the wrong decision, should I have returned home to Texas where I would have had support not only for me but also for my children.

> *"Even there Your hand will lead me, And*
> *Your right hand will lay hold of me."*
> *Psalm 139: 10 (NASB)*

The rest of that day's events are still cloudy in my mind, all I can remember was climbing into bed that night. I remember thinking, "What am I going to do? What am I suppose to do? Where am I going to go? Do I leave or stay? What is to come? Why would he leave, I thought we were working through all of his extracurricular marital activities." I can still feel the burden of all of the responsibilities being placed upon my shoulders that night. Fear had not yet set in, because I was still in disbelief. I had not yet comprehended the realness of it all. My heart and my life had not yet felt the piercing sting from the tip of the blade of rejection, only its glare from the shine was what I was experiencing.

Days would pass and I would spend a lot of time praying and crying and praying about crying, and asking God to make me stop crying. I was so tired of crying, my heart was aching, I missed my husband, but at the same time, I was so angry with him.

The pain of rejection along with the intentional betrayal was so intense that I could feel it physically. It felt as if a big part of me was savagely being ripped away with a jagged knife. According to the Bible (Mark 10:8 NIV: "for two will become one flesh. So they are no longer two, but one flesh."), half of me was indeed being torn away when my husband willfully abandoned us, I believe, without remorse.

I wanted nothing more than to have the agony from it all stop. The torment that resulted from the betrayal and lies made me desire death more than anything.

When the security of being with someone you love so much is stolen from you, it leaves a deep empty hole within you. The emotions of anger, betrayal, fear, misery, anxiety, brokenness, mistrust, confusion, discouragement, and depression is all that is left to fill those holes.

"If a man vows a vow to the Lord, or swears an oath to bind himself by a pledge, he shall not break his word. He shall do according to all that proceeds out of his mouth."
Numbers 30:2 (ESV)

I was with my husband for literally half of my life, which caused me to believe that my identity and who I was came from whom he was. We had grown into adulthood together, worked through so many good and bad things together, dreamed so many dreams together, but more importantly, we had made vows to each other; promising to take care of each other always, to support each other no matter what, and to always find a way to work things out together. My husband chose not to keep the vows he made to me though I still planned on keeping mine even after finding out about all of his unprotected extra marital activity during his most recent deployment to the Middle East and with Ema.

The mail came in and my husband's military credit card bill was in it. Something in my gut said to open it up. On the bill were two charges; one to a very well known hotel and the other was for dinner at an expensive upscale restaurant in San Diego. I called the hotel and the restaurant to get both the hotel folio and the dinner receipt using my power of attorney; both businesses fulfilled my requests. On the hotel folio, it listed very clearly the guest's names, those belonging to both my husband and Ema. Not only was Ema's name listed as the other person staying in the same room with my husband but her hotel rewards membership number was too. It also revealed that both of their confirmation numbers matched, their check-in and checkout times were exactly the same and that the one king size bed was reserved for the two of them. The dinner receipt showed exactly what they both had eaten as well as the name of the waitress who served them. I was livid, not only because I had begged my husband many times to take me to a nice hotel to get away, but the majority of my anger came from him having spent $500 for the entire evening and $200 of it on dinner alone, while he allowed our children and I to go hungry. He did not only refuse to give me enough money to survive but went on to threaten my life if I were to withdraw any money from our joint bank account. The amount of money he spent in one night on himself and Ema, would have fed our children and I for a month with money to spare.

This documented proof was not only my confirmation of Ema's existence but the revelation that my husband had not only lied to me but discarded us, his family, for some woman who did nothing to support him in any way for the last nineteen years. This truth plunged the blade of rejection deep into my heart and instantly destroyed the hope that filled it. I literally fell over in pain from the truth that had always resonated in my gut. I couldn't believe my husband had gone against everything he once stood for; honor, integrity, commitment etc. He didn't just betray me with this female, he didn't just disrespectfully lie to me, he didn't just break all of his promises, not just to me but to our children, he didn't just destroy all of our planned dreams and goals or strip me of all of my security but he abandoned me. He rejected our children. He rejected me.

As rejection stabbed my heart, pain poured out of it and hate began to fill it.

* * * * * * * * * * * * * * * * * * * *

In the Bible, there are many stories about rejection and betrayal. Joseph, one of my favorite people whom I share a similar story with is found in the book of Genesis. Joseph was rejected and betrayed by his beloved brothers when they sold him as a slave to Potiphar, one of Pharaoh's officers. Taken to Egypt against his will and unable to change his situation, Joseph, decides to become the best servant he could be; loyal, honest and hardworking. One day, Potiphar's wife attempts to seduce Joseph but he denies her, her embarrassment causes her to go to her husband with false accusations about Joseph. Potiphar believing the lies has Joseph thrown immediately into jail. While in jail, Joseph becomes friends with a fellow inmate, Pharaoh's official cupbearer. The cupbearer is soon released and Joseph asks that he remember

Joseph once he's released from jail. The cupbearer said he would, but failed to keep his word to Joseph.

If you have been rejected, then you can understand how Joseph must have felt when his own blood brothers whom he loved dearly, discarded him and then lied to their father about his disappearance; not only betraying him but stealing his life as well as his father from him. Then, after choosing to be supportive and loyal to Potiphar, Potiphar too, rejects Joseph believing the lies of his wife with no regard to Joseph's word, allegiance or their thirteen year history together.

Jesus, like Joseph was also rejected, as it is written in the Book of Luke, by His own people in His hometown of Nazareth. To the Nazarenes, Jesus always preached to them, healed them, and blessed them yet they still rejected Him. Then, in the book of John, Jesus is rejected and betrayed by two of his own disciples, Judas and Peter.

"The righteous cries out, and the Lord hears them; He delivers them from all of their troubles. The Lord is close to the broken hearted and saves those who are crushed in spirit."
Psalm 34:17-18 (NIV)

Like Joseph, I did not only feel rejected by the person I loved the most on this earth but I felt rejected and neglected also by my Potiphar, the military. My husband was a U.S. Marine, he was a good Marine and he was very good at what he did. I supported him from the time he was a young enlisted Lance Corporal, through his time as a decorated Sniper and up through the officer ranks of Marine Gunner. I not only helped him study for tests, do things to help make his life and job easier (iron his uniform, pack him lunches, send him care packages and letters when he was deployed, stopped everything I was doing to make his needs my priority, do his job at home when he couldn't or wasn't there, I held down the home front, Etc.) but I supported and served the Marine Corps for nineteen years as a semper fidelis Marine Corps wife, I supported Marines that I did not know personally as a patriotic American. The Marine Corps was the family that encompassed our family. When I found out about my husband and Ema I went to the people that were suppose to help me (Ema was a Marine Corps Captain) begging for their help. Asking them to make my husband and Ema stop cheating and to stop hurting our family but I was rejected. I was discarded and turned away and told that they would not help me. In essence, I was told that they were going to protect their Marine and more importantly their reputation as a whole, though it went against everything the Marine Corps stood for (honor, courage, and commitment), even though it went against the rules of the UCMJ (Uniform Code of Military Justice) and after learning that the people who were suppose to help me were "Christian" both parties chose to go against the beliefs of what us Christians believe about marriage and adultery. I felt betrayed not only my husband, but by the military branch of service that I served and loved for literally half of my life and even by Ema, a Marine that I supported though I did not know her when I chose to serve the Corps faithfully, Semper Fidelis-ly.

I once again felt alone, used, and discarded with no support from the people who were suppose to support me and who for nineteen years always said, "We take care of our Marine families because our Marines couldn't do what they do without them." Whose motto was "We never leave a man behind." and who stood for the idea of "We defend those who can't defend themselves." Words that I believed in with every part of me, words that I would and did live by, and words that I trusted and thought included me. In the end, they were just words, words that fed the power and the intensity of the pain I felt when I learned that I had been lied to, I had been betrayed, and once again, I had been rejected.

* * * * * * * * * * * * * * * * * * *

The truth is we have all been rejected; by someone, some group, or something at some point in our lives. Anytime anyone feels rejected, especially by somebody that is precious and important to him or her they're left devastated.

Rejection is one of the many wounds inflicted upon our heart that takes the longest time to heal from because its laceration cuts so deep. It is the most painful and powerful bondage that can be inflicted upon us, it is something we cannot see or touch but remains the strongest feeling we can feel and it has the ability to hinder us in every area of our life. Rejection is the strongest and the most devastating of all emotions because it slices straight to the core of the very person we are as well as what we think and feel about ourselves. Rejection isn't only an agonizing feeling but it sends a very influential and damaging message straight to the heart saying to us; "You are not worthy, you do not fit in, you do not belong, you are not good enough, I don't want you." Rejection leaves us questioning our worth, our value, and our purpose while creating a vicious cycle of destruction that causes us to become overly self-critical, it encourages us to wallow in self-pity, it demolishes our self-image, and shakes the very foundation of our self–confidence. Rejection causes us to believe lies about ourselves, provoking us to project upon other people thoughts about us that are not true, but more detrimental, rejection undermines our relationship with God. The crux of rejection is very powerful and difficult to recover from alone.

> *"The Lord is close to the brokenhearted and*
> *saves those who are crushed in spirit."*
> *Psalm 34:18 (NLT)*

Having been married to my husband for literally half of my life, practically growing up together, we shared all of life's biggest milestones together (we had our babies, started our family, bought our homes etc.) and we created dreams together; he was my best friend. Somewhere along the way I lost who I was and allowed my identity to be found in him. When he rejected me, I felt like a lost puppy that once had a home but was discarded and thrown away, left abandoned on the side of the road alone to find a new home on my own. I still feel like this from time to time and to be completely honest, I do get scared sometimes and I am unsure of my future but I take confidence and great courage in knowing that though I do not know what is to come, God does. As I sit here and write to you, I am not completely healed from the rejection that my husband forced upon my heart, my mind, and my soul, but I do know that I am closer to healing more now than I was. The wounds I carry from my husband are not yet 100% mended and may never be completely healed but they are definitely scabbed over, and they still bleed once in a while when he does things that are hurtful, but I have God who quickly binds them up for me. I know I am closer to healing because I am now courageously willing to trust and love others again with reckless abandon even knowing there is the possibility of being rejected again. I choose to love and to trust others again because I know that I get but one life. This is not to say I don't guard my heart (Proverbs 4:23) but I have come to realize that **we do only get one chance at life.** Knowing this fact, I refuse to allow my life or my heart to be filled with misery, bitterness, anger, resentment, or hurt because of the rejection I receive from others and I definitely don't want my heart to harden, keeping love from flowing in and out of it.

* * * * * * * * * * * * * * * * * * *

I want to share that it is healthy to take some time and grieve over your losses but to overextend the time is a detriment to your life. You must take the time needed to cry, to be sad, to ask God why, to be angry, and to cry some more. However, do not allow the grieving process to overtake your life, especially for a very long period of time. The more you allow rejection to defeat you, the longer and further it will carry you away from healing. This is not to say that you should just get over it, but while you go through the emotions and stages of grief, you need to make it a priority to work towards your healing. If you do not intently move towards healing, you will be persecuted by the adverse effects from its infliction; you will do one or many unhealthy and non productive things, such as; becoming rebellious or defiant, becoming a people pleaser, allowing your heart to become hard and filled with jealousy, blame, unforgiveness, envy, bitterness, and even hate, or a combination of any of these things. You will become someone you are not, desiring to be accepted, to feel loved by another or you may do the opposite and use others to get what you need. You may reject others because you are afraid of being hurt and rejected again, contributing to the vicious cycle of hurt. You will second guess yourself and question your worth. You will become overly sensitive and unable to receive constructive criticism, you will always feel the need to prove your worth to others, you will be unable to stand up for yourself because of the fear of conflict or confrontation and the fear of not being accepted for your thoughts, opinions, or rights. In short, you will become a victim.

How you react and respond to rejection will determine the life you lead and the outcome of your journey upon this earth. Dwelling on the misfortunes and the mistreatment done to us, does not help us because we cannot change it. It happened, it's over, go through the emotions but then learn from it, grow from it, be stronger because of it, choose to be a better person. I want to encourage you to choose life (Deuteronomy 30:15), choose healing (Psalms 147:3), choose peace (Philippians 4:7), choose freedom (Isaiah 61:1), choose what God is offering you (Isaiah 41:10); that which no other can offer.

"Then they cried to Lord in their trouble, and He
saved them from their distress. He sent forth
His word and healed them; He rescued them from the grave."
Psalm 107:19-20 (NIV)

I also want to encourage you to seek God as I did, allow Him to bind up your wounds. Go through the grieving process but do not stop living. Take time to cry, to question your situation for a short period, to go through the emotions but make a decision to want healing in the end, to want a life filled with happiness, and a life filled with peace, in summation, freedom from the bondage that rejection entwines you with. You only get one life, do not waste it! Remember also, you are not the only person who has or is going through what you are going through, though it may feel like it.

I want you to know, that though you have been rejected, **you are still loved and wanted by God**. (Romans 8:35) Find placidity in knowing that if I can get through my heart breaking pain, you can too. God helped me, and **God can and will help you! He <u>wants</u> to help you!** God finds you worthy, deserving and He sees you as precious and valuable. God is there to give you everything you need and He wants to love you the way you deserve to be loved. **God loves you. Do not deprive yourself of the love you are worthy of. You are loveable, worthy, important, and precious to God.** (Isaiah 43:2) Remember, your value doesn't decrease just because somebody else does not see your worth. People may not always see the treasures God has placed within you, so don't put too much value on their opinion. Trust that God knows what's in you and He will always choose you even when others overlook you. (Jeremiah 1:5)

The theme or title of my life really should be Rejection, not only because my husband rejected me but, because I have had so many people whom I care about reject me but my life's theme by the grace of God is not that of rejection. Rather, because of God, I have a life themed REDEMPTION and **you're life's theme can also be titled REEDEEMED!** If you so choose...

Chapter 2

CHOOSE

*"This day I call the heavens and the earth as witness
against you that I have set before you life and death,
blessings and curses. Now choose life..."*
Deuteronomy 30:19 (NIV)

Happiness, like LOVE, is not a state of being; it is a decision.
It is a choice given to us through free will. Feelings are fleeting,
they come and they go. They can change at any given moment, so
with that fact alone, you must always follow truth and not your
feelings. You must constantly and relentlessly believe truth and
not your feelings. Allow me to share with you a non-changing
fact that you must always remember as truth, especially in your
loneliest, darkest, most desperate moments...**what is true in the
light is still true in the dark.**

Your mind controls your body, your feelings, your choices, and
your decisions. So in order to be led by truth you must first conquer
your mind. Think about it, how do you become depressed, finding
yourself in complete hopelessness and defeat? Both hopelessness
and defeat emanates from the inability to control or guard your
thoughts. Rather than choosing positive, faith-filled thoughts,
you have allowed your feelings to control your mind and **when**

you allow your feelings to guide you, you will be misguided every time.

Going through my separation with my husband and for some time after, I fell into a depression. I allowed the "why" questions to saturate my mind and I permitted the guidance of my feelings of insufficiency to overtake my thoughts. The more I dwelt on those negative and self-defeating thoughts the more I believed them and soon I started to become them. I had allowed myself to become a victim and the more I meditated, if you will, on the damaging thoughts, for many hours of each day, the more of a victim I became filled with hopelessness. Before I knew it, I no longer had any self-worth, self-confidence, my self-esteem was non existent, and I had no desire to even live because I believed I was no longer valued or appreciated by the man who promised to never leave me and swore to work through every situation we would ever encounter. His lies, his rejection, his betrayal, his broken promises were the catalyst that initiated my self-destructive thoughts. The anguish caused from his destructive choices harmed my emotional state so severely, that the effects from it forged my feelings and my feelings led me into a downward spiral. Looking back now, I understand that I was wrong when I allowed his choices to effect me with such detriment. The price I paid for investing who I was in my husband cost me dearly. The short sightedness of my investment choice positioned me for bankruptcy in all areas of my life.

You should never allow or give any one person that much control or power over you. You should never let someone else's hurtful choices to influence you or impact your life that significantly. You should never place your identity and your worth in another person. **You were given the right** when we were born **to choose** the **life** you want, to be the author of your own life's story, not anyone else. Any person who is given the privilege to be in your life should be a compliment to your life <u>not</u> the center of it.

When I naively gave up my own identity for my husband's and made him the center of my life, I lost who I was and I made myself vulnerable to the devastation I endured. My husband's choice to leave me happened but it may not have been as traumatic to me had I kept my identity in God instead of having placed it in him. When he left, I was not only lost but I no longer knew who I was because I didn't own my identity; over the years, I had become his wife, our children's mother, and a wife of a Marine. I, Alysia no longer existed.

When I finally realized the extent of my loss, my hurt turned into anger…

> *"Stronger than lover's love, is lover's hate.*
> *Incurable, in each, wounds they make."*
> *- Euripides, Medea*

With each day that passed during my separation, and with each moment I was witness to my husband's rendezvous with his mistress, revenge became more inviting and intoxicating. I wanted nothing more than for the truth to come out and to be justified, I wanted someone to fight for me and for what I was fighting for—my family. But nobody would, not my husband, not the Marine Corps, not even other family members. I felt alone, scared, desperate, and bullied. I can remember going through the emotions of revenge as if it was only yesterday. The revenge, hatred, hurt, and pain that my heart felt left me wanting everything and anything dreadful to come to my husband and his sidekick Ema. I can remember wishing they would each die a painful death if not live the most miserable unproductive painstaking life upon this earth. I hurt so bad from the lies and the betrayal the two of them bestowed upon me and from the pain I watched my children endure because of their father's selfish choices created a strong yearning for my husband and Ema to feel the very pain they caused me in the deepest parts of my soul. My heart was consumed with so much hate and anger that my body temperature literally would rise at the very thought of them or the remembrance of the betrayal. I couldn't sleep at night and if I did sleep I would wake up at all hours throughout the night. My days were filled with thoughts of things I could or should have done and unproductive thoughts of things I should do. My righteous anger allotted me communication with Ema one time via text message when she had the audacity to ask me to not contact her parents after I had called her mother asking for her mother's support in protecting my family. Ema was too cowardly to face me or to even respond to my many requests to leave what was rightfully mine alone, my husband and to stop hurting our family. I wanted to let the world know what type of people Ema and my husband really were because they weren't the people they were claiming to be as they counterfeited behind their Marine Corps titles. As evidence proved they were far from being noble or ethical Marine Officers who represented honor, courage, and commitment.

"No temptation has overtaken you except what is common to man; but God is faithful, He will not allow you to be tempted beyond what you are able, but with the temptation, He will make a way, so that you can endure it." 1 Corinthians 10:13 (NIV)

The coinciding of my heart with wanting to do what God wanted always had a stronger pull, although minuscule, the indwelling pull was a bit more powerful than the tempting pull derived from hate. Though it was extremely difficult and emotionally draining, I chose to fight resolutely between the innate need to justify my feelings and the obedient choice to follow God's way. I did not gossip about them to others but if I am going to be quite honest, I did speak and communicated badly to my husband. I would degrade him for his selfish choices, I would emasculate him when he would not do right, and I would demean him when he would hurt our children or me and I would call Ema ungodly names when I spoke about her to him. The words that spewed out of my mouth fountained from my broken injured heart. (Matthew 12:34)

I can recount telling my husband exactly what I felt about what he and this female did to me, our children, our family, and I made sure it was very colorful and detailed. I was beyond frustrated and impatient with waiting and hoping he would do what was right, to do what I knew he once believed and was capable of doing, and to do it for the love he had for our children. But he was too weak to be the man he once was, the man I had known him to be. I was angry that he was failing us and himself and I was furious that he had changed the way I looked at him as a person and that his actions caused me to no longer respect him and I saw him as a coward. I was disappointed that he had become everything he once stood boldly against and I was the most resentful that he would allow our children to go through the heartache they were going through. I heartbreakingly remember when our youngest daughter tried to "negotiate" with him. She said to him, "Daddy, why don't you just stay, then four people will be happy and then you will be happy." His immediate and selfish answer to her was, "I need to be happy." How dare he choose his happiness over his very own child's heart, how dare he subconsciously speak to her heart telling her she wasn't worth the fight and that the female was loved more than her, how dare he tear away her security, how dare he discard our baby and our other two children with no regard or remorse. He was supposed to be the protector of their hearts yet he was the assailant who was destroying it along with their identity and he was gambling and risking the outcome of who they were to become. Employed and selected by God to be their mother and the other protector of their hearts I was enraged with a deep sense of loathing for their father, my husband.

I had had enough of being used, manipulated, and bullied by my husband and Ema and I was done with his abuse to our children's identities, hearts, and spirits. I was tired of hearing him constantly compare me to this female, informing me that she was better than me in every way while reminding me that she was now the choice of his life and I was tired of him spending and wasting our money on her. It was extremely difficult for me to act like a Christian is suppose to act when all I would hear and feel from him where his depreciating words that constantly assaulted and tore down my self-esteem, my self-worth, my heart, and my spirit. With each of his attacks upon my heart and mind the faster the hope and love I had inside of my heart emptied and refilled with hurt; hurt that turned into anger, anger that soon became hate and with that hate came the destruction of who I was at my core; my mind, my life, my words, and my spirit. My actions and thoughts began to permeate with rage, chaos, hopeless pain, bitterness, misery, and emptiness. My husband's self-centered selfishness stole my life, my happiness, and my peace not to mention the damage he inflicted upon the hearts and minds of our children was too much to bear and I wanted nothing more than to have my husband and Ema's consequences fall upon them in a mighty and savage way, this destructive desire outweighed wanting peace in my heart.

"Everyone who calls on the name of the Lord will be saved."
Romans 10:13 (NIV)

Finally weak, broken, emotionally fickle and practically non-existent, having nothing left, I fell before God begging for His help and asking for His forgiveness; for speaking ungodly once again towards my husband, and "pre-apologizing" because I knew that I was not disciplined enough to refrain from withholding my tongue when I would speak to my husband again. The pain that resonated within me overpowered any self-control I was supposed to have with my mouth. I did not only ask God for forgiveness and admitted to my faults but I shared my angry heart and adamantly informed God that I was holding Him to the promises He made me. I was weak and at times I felt possessed with the temptation to give into the consuming hate that was so strong within me. The battle between good and evil that raged within me was treacherously painful and exhausting, good barely won over the evil that was trying to consume me.

> *"Blessed is the man who remains steadfast under trial,*
> *for when he has stood the test he will*
> *receive the crown of life, which God has*
> *promised to those who love him."*
> *James 1:12 (ESV)*

Allow me to take you on a very important tangent; "No temptation has overtaken you except such as is common to man; but God is faithful, who will not allow you to be tempted beyond what you are able, but with the temptation will also make the way of escape, that you may be able to bear it." (1 Corinthians 10:13 NASB) This Scripture teaches us a powerful principle. If we belong to Him, **God will not allow any difficulty to come into our lives that we are not capable of bearing and He will always make a way for us to choose to get out, an escape.** God has say-so over everyone and everything in both the natural world and in the spiritual realm; He is in control of all things. (Luke 12:22-26) NOTHING, good or bad in our lives can happen to us or come upon us without God's permission. Even Satan, the adversary of both God and man, must go before God to ask if he can commit evil, place burdens or inflict pain upon us or within our lives. This is confirmed in the story of Job when Satan goes before God asking God to remove His protection around Job: "One day the angels came to present themselves before the LORD, and Satan also came with them" (Job 1:6 NIV) Satan inquired about and requested the removal of God's hedge of protection on Job's life. (Job 1:9-11 NIV) "The LORD said to Satan, "Very well, then, everything he has is in your hands, but on the man himself do not lay a finger." Then Satan went out from the presence of the LORD." (Job 1:12 NIV)

> *"I have said these things to you,*
> *that in me you may have peace. In the world you will have*
> *tribulation. But take heart; I have overcome the world."*
> *John 16:33 (ESV)*

When we were growing up we each had an idea or a dream of what we wanted our lives to be or be like; we had a goal and a plan to go with it, we could see and imagine how we wanted to live our lives and we knew who or how we wanted to be. Still today, we may have dreams or an idea about our lives. Like an unfinished book, the only things we are able to see and know are the parts of our life; the chapters, that have already transpired and the chapter, we are currently in. We tend to forget to remember, that which we are working towards, and we often forget that tomorrow is never promised to us. (James 4:14-15).

Right now, during these times of hurt and loneliness, remember that though this part of your life makes no sense at all, know that **God doesn't make any mistakes.** I want to reassure you that God knows dreams, your battles, or if you even get a tomorrow. He also knows your heart and all of its intricacies; the state it's in, it's desires and it's struggles. He has already designed and written his plan for your life, down to the smallest details. God never said we would understand everything that happens along the way, He didn't say we wouldn't have loss, pain, disappointment, setbacks, or heartaches but God did promise that it will all work out for our good. (Romans 8:28) So take confidence in knowing although you do not know the ending of your book or where your path will lead throughout the upcoming chapters, God has already written the final chapter. He knows what is to come, He knows the choices you will make with your free will, and more importantly, He knows how to carry you, guide you, and help you get to the last chapter of your book, your life. (Job 14:5) And know assuredly that you do get to help write the story of your life.

Remember, the pain you are going through is only one section, maybe only a chapter in your book and like the past chapters of your life, this chapter will also end and a new one will begin soon or later. This chapter that you are currently in may have nothing beautiful about it and may be extremely painful but it does pose an opportunity to <u>choose</u> between two options, two possible outcomes and YOU get to <u>choose</u> to write the next chapter. One that either continues with suffering or one that chooses to write a life's story that trusts God.

An unchangeable fact is; **this chapter of your life is needed and necessary to complete the entire story of your life** and when you reach the final chapter, all of this will come together and will make sense leaving the last chapter of your book as the end to an amazing story. The choices you make from here on out will decide whether your storybook of your life has a happy or a sad ending. Either way, it's the ending to the story of your life, the story <u>you</u> get to write. You are the co-author and the pen is in your hand.

"Everything in your life is a reflection of a choice you made.
If you want a different result, make a different choice."
- Anonymous

It is simply an unavoidable part of life that we all must experience pain in one time or another and undeniably we all have things that we just don't understand, having to go through and experiencing the pain from disappointments, setbacks, failures, and losses. More often than not, we easily get discouraged and bitter while trying to figure out why the painful things we are going through are happening to us. One reason is we can't see our futures and we don't know the destiny God has planned for our lives. (Jeremiah 29:11)

Inevitably pain will change you; heartaches and losses never leave you the same. This chapter you are in will end and you will get to the next one hopefully, sooner than later, but no matter the time it takes to get to the next chapter, at the end of this chapter, you will definitely be different. How the pain changes you is up to you. You can either choose to come out of your situation bitter, defeated, quitting on your dreams and life goals, resenting life, the people in it and God or you can come out better, stronger and more trusting of God (Proverbs 3:5-6) with freedom and a new passion being on fire, excited about writing the next chapter of your life.

Recognize that **pain is always an opportunity to become stronger**, to gain a new confidence, to develop more character, to learn new things about yourself, and to discover the strength and limits within you. It's always easy to give up, but I want to encourage you to keep fighting, to keep holding on, and to keep hoping and not allow what you are going through to overwhelm you. I boldly ask that you do not allow the pain you are enduring to be in vain. God did not permit the pain, difficulties, heartaches and losses you endure to hurt you or to stop you but rather, to prepare you, increase you, develop you, transform you, and to propel you forward to greater things. (1 Peter 5:10) Remember, **God is in control** of our lives and the lives of our enemy. God is the potter, (Isaiah 64:8) the sculptor, and the designer and if the pain were going to harm you instead of help you He would not have let you gone through it. The fire you are enduring may be excruciatingly hot but know that God has allowed it because you are strong enough to get through it; all you have to do is hang on and trust God.

Know that **the God who breathed life into you, also crowned you with favor; He takes pleasure in prospering you, He is for you and not against you** (Romans 8:31) and is in complete control of all things as He still and forever will reign upon his throne. <u>Choose</u> to not be a whiner, but instead a warrior that fights through it so that you will come out increased, promoted and better than you are. You have heard of the saying, "No pain no gain." Realize that every struggle that you endure in your life is to make you stronger, every difficulty is to grow you up, and every painful time is there to develop something in you that can only be developed in the most painful times. (Romans 5:3) If everything were always easy you wouldn't be prepared for your destiny. If you stay in faith, you will be led to your destiny. Don't just go through your hard and painful time; instead grow through it and remember that experience is the best teacher.

Finally, if you choose to come out better God has an amazing plan where He will use your life to be a light for others who need that light in their dark times. I can testify to this, because I sit here writing to you in hopes that all of my pain, heartache, and loss will give you comfort, hope, encouragement, or even be a shimmer of light at the end of your dark tunnel. I hope to be an inspiration to you, encouraging you to write an amazing end to your life story.

* * * * * * * * * * * * * * * * * * * *

"So then each one of us will give an account of himself to God."
Romans 14:12 (NASB)

I know that God already knew what choices I would make. It was extremely hard to choose the higher ground every time, the path less traveled as it often is, and many times, I confess, I did not choose the higher ground especially when it came to interacting with my husband, for two reasons: First, because the feelings and the love I had for my husband ran so deep that it made the pain he inflicted upon me more concentrated; and second, I didn't know what God's truths were at the time, making it harder to turn the other cheek or to choose right. (Matthew 5:39, Luke 6:29) God warns in Hosea 4:6 that when we don't know His word, we will be destroyed. This is true and I learned the hard way. Our, both my husband and my lack of knowledge of God's word during our marriage paved the path to the destruction of our unity. I can look back and see that it was only by God's grace that I was able to endure and overcome, but more importantly, the lessons I learned from the fall of my marriage are now tattooed upon my heart. It was only by God's love for me that I learned what the true meaning of love (1 Corinthians 13:4-8) was. God loved me so much that He allowed my world to come crashing down, I will go more into depth on this in a later chapter.

"All things, work together for the good for those who love Him,
and are called according to His purpose."
Romans 8:28 (NIV)

God kept his Romans 8:28 promise to me. He used all of the bad things that have happened to me to cause me to look inward at myself, to see the things that I needed and wanted to change so that I would change and transform into a better person, a person who will and who is fulfilling my purpose upon this earth. From my brokenness I learned to speak kindly and to always act in love even during a disagreement and to not be led by my emotions but by truth especially in the hardest times. I am not claiming to have walked confidently in truth every single time I had a disagreement with my husband or with anyone but I have grown for the better since the point of betrayal and I thank God that I'm not where I use to be. My husband however, like me, lacked the knowledge shared in God's word and so the mistreatment I endured from him was very painful. I understand that hurt people hurt but the degree to which I was hurt and the things he put me through was on another level.

Ignorance and lack of knowledge of God's word, is never an excuse or a crutch to enable or justify any one person's bad choices.

> *"Accountability breeds response-ability."*
> *- Stephen Covey*

The choices I made when I chose to do wrong; reacting not in love, acting from a place of anger, speaking words filled with poison etc. throughout my marriage and through my divorce though I may have been justified in the natural, the choices I made were still wrong. These wrong choices, though at times seemed small and insignificant were the little foxes (Solomon 2:15) as the bible refers to them, that tore away the core of our marriage and because I, like my husband, made those small destructive choices, we also ignorantly and inadvertently chose, the outcome. I am not taking full responsibility of the division between my husband and I; please do not think that I am. He like me was wrong, he was extremely wrong and he too often made many harmful and erroneous choices. Though his detestable choices were a major component of our breakdown, I can only take responsibility and accountability for my part.

You too will **need to take responsibility and accountability for your transgressions,** especially **if you want to move forward.**

It was when I chose to face my misdeeds and dealt with the inner dark parts of my heart and my brokenness that I was able to learn, let go, and begin to heal and to grow. I had to choose to do what most fear, and that was to take a good hard look at who I was, who I had become, and realize why I had become it. Yes, many bad things happened to me as a child which caused me to carry baggage, if you will, into my marriage, and yes many bad things were inflicted upon me by my husband and many others during my marriage as well as throughout my life, but what it came down to, were MY choices. My choices that led to my outcome and to the person I had become, the person, once I took a hard look at, I did not like.

"It is better to offer no excuse than a bad one."
- George Washington

Many people will use their past as a crutch, an excuse and even as justification for their bad choices; I did it unconsciously and at times consciously. But I have come to learn that I could not and cannot rightfully say or justify that my past tribulations resulted in the present choices I made: I screamed and yelled because that was how I was communicated to, I threw things because I watched my parents do it, hence, I was abusive because I grew up in an abusive home leaving me ignorant and unaware to the proper or healthy way of converting my emotions into words.

Although those things happened to me, despite the fact they are understandable explanations, they were nonetheless not viable excuses or justifications for my choice to react and act in unproductive and unloving ways when I was frustrated, angry or hurt. During those moments of despair, I still had a choice in the way I chose to act and react. It would be wrong to use any of my past misfortunes and afflictions as my crutch, my reason, my excuse and certainly not my justification for the times I responded ill-mannered, unkind or coarse to any one person.

As for my husband, his childhood left him missing parts of a whole as well and yes he had fought in a war zone more times than he or anyone needs to, but in the end, it was still not enough to be used as a crutch, an excuse, something to hide behind or a free pass to get away with the unacceptable behavior nor a reason for not choosing right.

It is absolutely not fair or right to use the bad things that happened to you as an excuse, a reason, a rationalization or even a justification as the explanation for your choices. What I am trying to say is that **the things that have hurt you are <u>NEVER</u> enough of a reason to hurt or wrong other people or to make bad choices.**

You may have been sexually violated as a child or as an adult, or physically abused, maybe even victimized emotionally, or you were witness to or unwillingly took part in any abuse, it still is not a rational reason for your choices. Yes it is very bad that any of it happened to you, I am very sorry that it did, I really am and you did not deserve it, but as harsh as this may sound, you are not the only one who has had those bad things happen to you. I don't mean to sound callous but I had someone say that to me when I was going through my separation and it hurt but there was truth to it. It feels like you're the only one going through the hurt you are enduring, but know that you are not. There are many who are going through it right now just as you are, and there are many who have already gone through it, some survived and others were defeated by it and sadly, there will be many who will go through the same torment after you. So like me, you do not have permission to use ANY of it as an excuse for why you do the things you do. **You are NOT a Victim. STOP using the things from your past as an excuse for why you are the way you are. You are the way you are because you CHOOSE to be that way.** You are not weak, just because you feel weak. God did not allow the events of your past to happen to you so that you could use the pain as a scapegoat, He allowed the things that have happened to you to make you stronger to make you an overcomer. It was you who chose to be a victim instead of being victorious. So I tell you this in love, if you truly want to be happy and you truly want freedom, and you seriously want to move forward, then look at the bad breaks, the calamity, and the painful sufferings you have endured and say, "Yes, that happened to me, yes, it hurt, yes I am angry from it, yes it was wrong, but it happened and I can not change it, I cannot get back what was lost, what was stolen from me (my innocence, my childhood, the time, etc.). However, I will choose to not take on the role of a victim. Instead, I will choose to learn from it, I will not do to others what was done to me, I refuse to be the continuation point of the lifeless cycle, I will not give it the power to control my emotions, my thoughts or my life, instead, I will use it to fuel my passion to do something great and I will stop this vicious cycle and not let it continue anymore." I WILL CHOOSE LIFE.

"Just as the Son of Man did not come to be served,
but to serve, and to give his life as a ransom for many."
Matthew 20:28 (NLT)

Jesus Christ, the Son of God sacrificed His life for you and me long before we ever knew of Him. Out of Jesus' infinite love for us, He died on the cross for yours and my sins so that we would not only have life everlasting but to give us a life that is filled with victory and freedom and peace while we walk upon this earth. He did not die for us to be victims, but rather to be victorious, to be overcomers and to be champions. Jesus died to give YOU life, a life to live in an extraordinary way. Jesus' death was too high of a price for Him to have had paid for us, the very least we can do is to choose to give honor for the selfless choice He made for our sake. Jesus doesn't ask for anything more than for you to accept Him, to profess that He is the Son of God, to love Him in return, to trust Him and to give Him all of your burdens and to choose Him and all that he freely offers.

"Carefully guard your thoughts because
they are the source of true life."
Proverbs 4:23 (CEV)

Throughout my separation and divorce, I was given many opportunities to make choices and decisions, choices and decisions that led to an action, and I can honestly say, the majority of them were hard to make. They were hard in terms of the right, the good, or the correct options were not always the easiest or the choices I wanted to make. The proper choice more often than not, opposed my feelings, which made it more difficult to want to choose it. So many times my husband would do something unkind to me, or say something very mean to me, or again reject me and our children and each time I had to choose how I was going to react or respond. I can honestly say I did not always make the best choice and I did not always respond in kindness or love. I share this with you because I don't want you to think that I am trying to portray myself as some saint, because I am not. I am a Christian but I am also a human with feelings; who is capable of being hurt and one who will stumble from time to time. I want to tell you that you too, will not always make the correct response when someone hurts you and I won't say that it's all right but I will say, it is understandable. **Hurt people hurt other people.** However, you, like I did will have to soon or later, the sooner the better, choose to respond in the manner that you would want to be responded to, had your situation been the other way. It is not only the mature thing to do but; the right thing to do and more importantly it is the key that <u>will</u> unlock you from the bondage that you are living in. It will lead you to freedom and healing.

All of our choices, whether good or bad, come with an outcome, either good or bad.

We are the only people we can control and we are the only ones who can and will be held accountable in the end for the choices (words, actions, deeds etc.) we make.

I share some intimate details of my heart, my life and from my marriage with you to testify, that even when someone mistreats you, abuses you, betrays you, lies to you, uses you, and hurts you; you still have a choice, **you always have a choice.**

Though I have suffered much pain and heartache I choose to live intentionally, on purpose. I could not allow the hurts to steal away the remaining years of my life, I couldn't let the people who hurt me win nor could I let everything my children or me endured to be in vain. I try to resolve issues with the people I have issues with, letting my pride go and always trying to seek to understand more than to be understood, and extending mercy, grace, and patience when I can because I know there will come a time that I will need it extended to me. I try to be humble with humility. I choose to love people with reckless abandon, living with a sense of crazy love and trying to love others in their own love language. One thing I can testify to is when God allows one person to be removed from my life no matter how painful it is He has always brought me two better people. I choose to be in the moment of every moment. I choose to walk in God's will for my life each day. I choose to be thankful for every little thing. I consciously make it a point to always have a heart filled with gratitude. I try my best to make the most of each day and to smile even when I am hurting. These things that I have chosen to do, I did not choose to do for the praises of people, but because the rewards that I get: a sense of happiness, a heart filled with joy, a life of purpose and the love that I get back is far greater than anything money could ever buy. I also choose these things because I serve an audience of One, I don't need the admiration of others to feel accepted or accomplished. In the end I am choosing to be happy and to walk in love in all aspects of my life because I want and I choose peace and freedom.

I share all that I have chosen to do with and in my life because I want you to understand that the place that I was emotionally, mentally, and spiritually is now a fading memory of my past. I share because if I can choose victory over the option of using my shortcomings, my disappointments, my failures, and my pain as excuses then you can too.

Before you can do anything, before you can move forward, closer to healing, to completeness, to happiness, you MUST choose. You must choose and decide right now in this very moment that enough is enough and that you are NOT a victim and you must refuse to be a victim. You must set your mind and your heart on victory, on wholeness, on peace. Jesus does not call us to be victims but rather overcomers. In John 5:1-15, Jesus tells the sick man who claimed to be a victim of passer-byers as he laid by the water for many years to pick up his mat and to walk. Jesus' words command us to not lie idly by the wayside, just allowing our lives to pass by us, hoping that someone would feel sorry for us and or our situation. Instead, to get up and fight for the things we want. You need to do the work that needs to be done for change and not wait or hope for someone else to do it for you. Talking about your situation to anyone and everyone all of the time in hopes that they are sympathetic towards you does not do anything more than just having someone listen to you complain about your hard knocks. It does not change your situation nor does it help your situation in any way.

Prayer however, leads to change. Change that requires action. Talk is not an action; it's simply just talk but there is power in prayer. So if you want change you must choose, you must then take action, and your first action should always be prayer.

Chapter 3

PRAYER

*"For you have been a stronghold to the poor, a
stronghold to the needy in his distress, a shelter
from the storm and a shade from the heat."*
Isaiah 25:4 (ESV)

What is prayer? It is an intimate conversation between you
and God. It's the time you share your heart, your fears, your
thoughts, your hurt, your wants, and your desires. It's where you
share your every thing with Him. Prayers to God can be done
in any language, at anytime of the day or in any place. You can
pray on your knees or standing up, you can pray with your eyes
open or shut, you can bow your head or not. Prayer is your time
with God. God is with you when you are alone, when you are in
your hardest times, when you think nobody cares or sees you
as well as being present in your good times. God is omnipotent
(all powerful), omnipresent (all present, He is everywhere), and
omniscient (all knowing, He sees and hears everything). **God is
with you everywhere you go.**

God is NOT surprised by ANYTHING you say, He already
knows. He just desires that you share it with Him and to spend
some intimate time alone with Him. When we pray, we not only
get closer to God but we invite Him to be present and to move in

our lives for us and for our situation. Prayer gives God permission to fight for you and on your behalf.

Every time you connect with God in prayer, you are praising Him because you are acknowledging your need to set your burdens on His strong shoulders. God takes care of His children (if you are not one of His children, I will share at the end of this book how you can become one if you do so choose), especially in the darkest part of the storm. He is there as a stronghold (Psalm 18:2) to keep you standing against the crashing waves and raging winds.

"Pour out your heart like water before the presence of the Lord"
Lamentations 2:19 (ESV)

God does not care if you yell at Him and tell Him how mad you are at the person or people who have hurt you, or if you tell Him you are mad at the world, or even that you are mad at Him. You can say to God, "I can't believe you let this happen, I am SO mad at you! I thought you loved me, I was a good Christian or a good person..."

I know this because I prayed these things. I literally yelled at God, I boldly and disrespectfully reminded Him of who I was and what I did for Him and on His behalf. I shared EVERYTHING and it wasn't the most polite or submissive or kind things.

"In my distress I called to the LORD; I cried to my God for help.
From his temple he heard my voice;
my cry came before him, into his ears."
Psalms 18:6 (NIV)

I prayed, as I stood in the shower as the hot water from the showerhead fell over me I stood firmly and yelled at God demanding that He tell me why this was happening to me. "Why would you God, allow my husband to walk away from us after being together for so long and through so much? Why did you,

God let it get to this point when I was "good; I was good to people; I was a good wife, a good mom, a good citizen in society, a good Christian, I was a good person and I don't deserve this, not any of it!" I screamed at God as an "entitled" victim. God began to answer me. As God spoke to me my anger and confusion turned into feebleness and I was no longer standing assertively with fists clinched. My body now leaned propped up against the shower wall, tears began to fall from my eyes as I stood their staring at the wall in front of me as God replayed my past, recollecting the events of our marriage and the recent months that had past. As my mind flipped through the photo album in my head God showed me who I was, who I had become. He showed me yelling, he showed me angry, he showed me impatient, he showed me frustrated, he showed me hurt, he showed me my heart and all of the darkness that had consumed it because I was no longer in control of my emotions. He showed me what I looked like when fear and anxiety dominated me. Watching the reel in my head caused my body to slide to the shower floor onto my knees, sadness and remorse flooded every part of my body. I began to bawl and throw up while I prayed because the sadness that I was feeling turned into unbearable pain. Rocking back and forth I felt ashamed, embarrassed, and heartbroken for the things I had done, for the ways I reacted, for the things I said. How did I allow myself to become so angry, so emotionally out of control, how and when did I give the hurt that was within me so much authority and power in and over my life? Sorry and regretful I now laid prone in the fetal position shaking and crying because my heart wouldn't stop bleeding from the pain that caused its wound as the now lukewarm water cascaded over my naked weak body. As the water from the showerhead fell upon my shaking body I poured out my heart to God as I begged Him to forgive me and to make the torment that I was feeling inside to stop. I sorrowfully apologized for the person I had become, for the resentment, bitterness, and anger I allowed to control me, and for my many unkind and immature reactions that did not come from love but rather from hurt, fear, and anger. I apologized for hurting the husband God had given to me and for the things I said and did that hurt; not only my husband but also; my children, our family, our marriage. I apologized to God for hurting Him as well. My heart was broken open, as I lay there remorseful acknowledging and taking accountability and responsibility for all of my wrong doings. I could feel the water turn cold but it was a cleansing feeling as I laid vulnerable and humble repenting of my transgressions to God. I noticed the quiet that now surrounded me, my cheek to the shower floor I noticed my breath had slowed down, I could feel my heartbeat in my chest, and I could hear the water run down the drain as it carried away all of misdeeds, shortcomings, offenses, and wrongdoings that I had just confessed to. God had just forgiven me and I could feel it from within, a burden had been lifted off of me, I felt light, I felt cleansed, though the water was now cold I felt God's presence come over me and I felt thankful for the undeserving grace God just covered me with, it was a feeling of comfort, and security, I felt free, no longer in bondage to the darkness that was overtaking my heart, and I had peace that surpassed all understanding. I could no longer hear or feel the chaos that was clamoring so loud within me, it was quiet, it was peaceful, and I was calm; it was nice.

Every single time I prayed or cried, God was there, listening. I want to share some of the prayers I prayed with you that helped God move in my life, prayers that began my healing and transformation spiritually, mentally, emotionally, and physically. I am not encouraging you to be disrespectful to God. I am simply sharing that having a personal relationship with God means you are free to be who you are; you are free to share your emotions at any volume level, you are free to speak your mind and what is in your heart, and you are free to be real, open, and vulnerable with no repercussions or judgments. God will simply listen, He will give you what you need and ask for according to his will and desire for you, He will move in a powerful way on your behalf when your heart is sincerely desiring him.

There is not a certain way to pray, prayer is not a ritual, it's not hard to do and prayer doesn't have to sound eloquent or even intelligent. Many get nervous when they pray and others have no clue how to pray. Prayer is simple. You just simply talk to God just like you are talking to any other person, preferably with some reverence but none the less, a simple conversation with God is prayer. You begin prayer by desiring to want to speak to God about any topic, any person or what is heavy on your heart. Once you have the desire, you then submit yourself to Him and you invite Him, asking Him to help you in any and all areas of your situation and or life. When you ask God you must trust that He is listening, trust that He wants to help you, trust that He is more than able to help you, trust that He has your very best interest at heart, and have faith that He will do what you ask when you believe that He can.

Remember: **A man/woman on his/her knees in prayer can stand before any tragedy.**

Here is one, of the many prayer I shared with God.

"Heavenly Father,

I am so angry right now. I am so scared; I don't know what to do, where to go, or what's going to happen. I need something but I don't even know where to start or what to ask for. I repent for the things I have done wrong, for being disrespectful to you and for the mean things I have said. Please show me what I need to repent for so that I can be clean before you, so You will hear my prayers but more so You can move in my life, in my situation, and in my heart. I pray this in Jesus' name. Amen."

This prayer God answered for me. He showed me what I needed to repent for. He didn't "care" about my situation what He cared about was the state of my heart and changing me for His glory.

Allow me to elucidate my conversation with God as I lay on the shower floor; God spoke to me and I attentively listened to Him. He reminded me of the things that I had done in my past that was ungodly. He gave me remembrance of my yelling at my husband, the destructive words I spoke, the slamming of doors and cabinets, the things I threw and He showed me the anger that derived from fear but was sin in my heart. God says in his Word, You can "be angry but do not sin." (Ephesians 4:26 ESV) I never understood what this verse meant until this moment.

> *"Man must evolve for all human conflict a method*
> *which rejects revenge, aggression, retaliation.*
> *The foundation of such a method is love."*
> *- Martin Luther King Jr.*

I can remember vividly; the revenge, the hatred, the hurt and the pain that my heart felt and all I wanted was everything and anything bad to come to my husband and Ema. I wished more than anything that they would both die a painful death if not live the most miserable unproductive painstaking life upon this earth. I hurt so bad and wanted them to feel the pain they caused in the deepest parts of my soul. My mind was consumed with so much hate and anger that my body temperature literally would rise at the very thought of it. But in the end my heart coincided with wanting to do what God wanted. Instead of speaking evil upon them I told God what I felt and told Him that I was holding Him to the promises He made me. This was my prayer:

"God,

I hate them so much. I wish they would both die. Why won't you kill them already? I don't know what is taking you so long to help me! I am SO angry at your slowness. You see me in pain and you and I both see them enjoying their lives together at the expense of my suffering and the suffering of my children and neither of them could care less. I hate them and God YOU promised me that you would avenge me! I WANT my revenge and please make it a slow and painful one for each of them and please let me watch."

Yes, that is not your typical, kind or even respectful prayer but it was the sharing of my true heart. I was so angry that God was taking His "sweet" time with vindicating me that I didn't even care that I was disrespectful to Him and I couldn't even bring myself to say amen at the end. I felt like a spoiled only child. I felt like He needed to give me exactly what I wanted at the exact moment I wanted it. My prayer was so full of rage that it was extremely passionate in the sense of all of me was dedicated to the words I prayed, my emotions were intense and every part of me was behind every single word that I spoke. If it were possible to see in the natural the physical force, strength and compelling hatred I had in those words you would have seen it move mountains literally. During this time the devil spoke into my heart. He also could see that I was full of hate, anger, and vengeance and tempted me to do things that would go against God. Part of me was very tempted. I knew in my heart of hearts that if I changed my prayers from God and gave my requests to Satan, not only would Satan do it but also he would delightfully do it and I would get to partake in the pleasure for a brief moment. The desire to enter into an agreement with the dark side was so powerful and ravenous that

I almost gave into it but wise enough to know that my choice to choose evil would return to me soon or later.

* * * * * * * * * * * * * *. * * * * *

God was more concerned with the state of my heart than He was with getting my revenge for me. He knew that I was dying inside and that if I continued on this path it would lead to my destruction and the loss of my destiny. Soon, my prayers began to change from angry prayers to prayers of desperation because I felt lost, I felt I was no longer in control, I was broken, I felt defeated and powerless. God's love for me allowed me to hit rock bottom because it was there that I had no other option but to cry out to Him for help. And so I did.

"God,

I can't do this anymore. I can't do this alone. I need your help. I am hurting. I don't know which way to go, where to go, or what to do. My heart is consumed with hate, hurt, and anger. I am dying, I feel lost, beat up, helpless and defeated. Please forgive me, help me to forgive the people who have hurt me and please help me to forgive myself. I give all of my pain to you and I ask that you replace it with your peace, your joy, and your wisdom. Help my unbelief when I doubt and please show me the hope my heart so desperately needs. Please take my brokenness and make it whole again. Heal me. Please give me beauty for my ashes as You promise. Let my tears turn into pure laughter. Make my life be a testimony that will help others later. In Jesus' name. Amen."

Again, it wasn't until I spent time in prayer that I was able to see my wrong doings. God reproducing images of those moments when my desperate reactions overtook me was not only a very painful experience however, one that was very much needed. Though, in the flesh my reactions one would argue, were justified but in God's eyes they were not, they did not respond in love as He had commanded. Just because my husband chose to break his word, or the many times he chose his friends over the kids and I and our scheduled family time, or even when he chose to give what was rightfully mine to other women, I still did not have the right to demean him with my words. It was those small foxes that aided in the destruction of our marriage. Yes I was right to be angry but to sin in anger was wrong. In that transparent moment with God I had to take accountability for my actions. I had to confess all of my lies, hurts, and offenses to God. I also chose to acknowledge the hurt I caused my husband during our arguments and throughout our marriage and I chose to admit to God that I was wrong. I chose to apologize, not just apologize but to apologize specifically; "I am sorry that I ____." I chose to ask for forgiveness. I chose to forgive my husband. I chose not to return evil with evil (1 Peter 3:9 & Romans 12:17) even after I learned about the attempts to slander my name and my character. I chose to seek understanding knowing my husband was deceived and hurt and out of deception he made his choices. The choices I chose despite his unkind actions towards me does not make me a better person than my husband, please know that is not what I am trying to convey but rather to let you know that I chose this path because I refused to allow my husband's hurtful choices towards me to steal any more of my freedom, my life or my peace. I am choosing the ending to my life's story and the outcome that I want.

Are you at a place where you're ready to choose but you just don't know how? You don't know how to guard your thoughts? Are you wondering how to take the higher ground, the path less traveled, when you're heart hurts so much? Especially when the hurt is deep, and your heart is heavy laden and the battering is new. Or your pain may not be fresh and raw and you may have been carrying the burden of it all for some time now. Either way, it's not too late to choose, **it's never to late to choose**, you can choose to stay and remain or you can choose to change and be free. Know though, **freedom is not free**, it is never free and it will require and it always will require, a sacrifice. Sacrifice demands an action however, remember; action invariably leads to change and change begins with prayer. If you are ready please pray the following prayer with your heart whether you know God or not. It's time to let go and let God.

> Lord God,
> I am lost. I am hurt. I am desperate. I don't know if you love me, I don't know if I matter but I do know that I need you. I need your help, I need what you have for me, I need to know you more, I need you to move in my life and on my behalf, I need you to fix my life and my heart. I can no longer do this alone and I am asking for your help. I have done wrong, I am wrong and I confess to you that I have _____ (fill in the blank with all of your misdeeds and shortcomings) and I am sorry. Please change my heart and make me better, make my life better. Change me from the inside out. Take my burdens and give me peace, joy, security, and love. Teach me to love like you do and to see others as you do. Help me to forgive others and myself as you forgive and help me to be kind to the people who have wronged me. Lead my mind and my life. Give me the words to speak and give me self-control. Let me fulfill my purpose, your will, on this earth and to live the life your son, Jesus Christ died to give me. I am sorry. I am

unworthy of your mercy and grace but I need it. Please come into my life and transform me, make me into the person you created me to be. Give me an abundant life and bless me so that I may be a blessing to others. Help me and heal me and fix all of the brokenness inside of me. Thank you Lord for listening to me, for hearing my prayer, and for moving in my life according to your will for it and for your forgiveness, mercy and grace. I receive all that you have for me. I pray all of this believing, in your son, Jesus' name. Amen.

HOW TO PRAY

- Praise God – Always begin your prayers praising God.

- Ask for forgiveness or ask to be shown what you need to ask forgiveness for.

- Pray for other people. This includes forgiving them or asking God to help you forgive them. Pray for their needs.

- Talk to God about your life and all that's happening. Ask Him for the things you need.

- Ask God to give you what He wants you to have. Ask for His will for your life.

- Thank God for all that you have.

Chapter 4

FORGIVENESS

*"To be a Christian means to forgive the
inexcusable because God has
forgiven the inexcusable in you." - C.S. Lewis*

Forgiveness is about personal power, about freedom. Forgiveness is for your benefit, not for anyone else. Forgiving the person who hurt you does not mean you have to reconcile with them and it does not mean you are condoning their behavior, it simply means you are choosing peace.

"Come out from among them and separate."
2 Corinthians 6:17 (MSG)

I, like David in 1 Samuel, had many justified reasons to seek revenge but like David, I did not. I did not because I needed to be forgiven so I forgave. I forgave so I could be free. ("Make allowances for each other's faults, and forgive anyone who offends you. Remember, the Lord forgave you, so you must forgive others." Colossians 3:13 NLT) I wanted to be free from the enemy and all of his strongholds ("Get rid of all bitterness, rage and anger, brawling and slander, along with every form of malice." Ephesians 4:31 NIV) and from the bondage and chaos that my life was consumed with. I did not want the enemy to gain anymore of a foothold in my life (Ephesians 4:27) because when he does, it always ends in destruction. Christ did not die for me to live a life full of bitterness and anger but one of victory. I chose not to be a victim but instead a conqueror. (Romans 8:37) I decided to let go and let God. (Psalm 55:22) Lastly, I chose to pray for my husband and even for Ema. I prayed for their relationship with God, for God to bring them godly people to speak truth into their lives and to remove all of the ungodly people in their lives that fed their sins, including themselves from one another's life. I prayed asking God to soften my husband's heart towards me, and I prayed that the Holy Spirit would convict both my husband and Ema's hearts and to give them revelation. I also prayed, if they willfully refused, like Paul prayed for his friends in 1 Corinthians 5:5, I prayed that they'd be delivered unto Satan for the destruction of their flesh for the saving of their souls. But more importantly, I chose to pray for myself. I asked God to give me the wisdom, the patience, the understanding, and the compassion I needed to get through all of this, to act the way I needed to towards my enemies and each situation, and to keep my heart right before Him. I asked God to show me what I needed to learn from all of this, to make me a quick learner and I also prayed for the healing of my heart. Lastly I prayed for forgiveness. I prayed for the strength to forgive not only my husband and I prayed for supernatural strength to be able to forgive Ema.

Prayer is an act of forgiveness. To pray for those who hurt you is an outwardly expression and request to God. It says, "I want to forgive, I want peace, I don't want the pain anymore, and I need God because I can not do it on my own."

"Life is hard and unfair. It is cruel and heartless, painful, trying, disappointing, unapologetic, and frequently downright awful. But that's not important. What's important is that through it all you learn how much you need your Heavenly Father..."
– Richelle E. Goodrich

Yes, life is hard and it's unfair that bad things happen to us, but God never said it would be easy, fair or even kind. We are living in a world that is in a battle of good versus evil. In this battle we are not able to control the things that other people do to us let alone what they say to us. The ONLY thing we can control is what we choose to do; how we act, how we react, how we think, the words we speak, the deeds we do and the actions we take.

> *Refrain from anger and turn from wrath;*
> *do not fret—it leads only to evil.*
> *Psalm 37:8 (NIV)*

No matter how bad something is done to you by another, it is not enough to justify you choosing to do wrong or paying them back for what they did to you. You may say, "But you don't know what he or she did to me, you don't understand." You may be right, I might not know what he or she did to you, or said to you, or said about you and I might not know or even understand the depth of the your pain, but God does. He also says to trust Him and to know not only will He turn this bad situation to good for those who love Him (Romans 8:28) but God also makes a promise to us in 2 Chronicles 16:9; that His eyes roam to and fro throughout the whole earth (this means He sees everything and He is all knowing, having all knowledge, understanding, and awareness) to show Himself strong on behalf of those who love Him, trust Him. God promises He will show Himself strong in our lives and in our situation(s) if we trust Him. God promises many times over that He will fight for you and on your behalf and avenge you to your enemies. "I will take revenge; I will pay them back. In due time their feet will slip. Their day of disaster will arrive, and their destiny will overtake them." (Deuteronomy 32:35 NLT). "Beloved, never avenge yourselves, but leave it to the wrath of God, for it is written, "Vengeance is mine, I will repay, says the Lord." (Romans 12:19 ESV). "And will not God bring about justice for his chosen ones, who cry out to him day and night? Will he keep putting them off?" (Luke 18:7 NIV). Not only does God promise to get your revenge upon your enemies, know that His revenge is far greater than any revenge you could give, but He promises to show your enemies how He has chosen you and then blesses you many times over because you loved Him, trusted Him, obeyed Him, was faithful to Him. "You prepare a table before me in the presence of my enemies. You anoint my head with oil; my cup overflow." (Psalm 23:5 NIV) As a child of God, you matter to Him and anyone that hurts you hurts God, you belong to Him and like a mother bear He will pay your offenders back for what they have done to you. "God is just; He will pay back trouble to those who trouble you..." (2 Thessalonians 1:7 NIV)

With all of this it is very important that you remember that with EVERY single choice that you make there comes with it an outcome, a consequence if you will. If you are willing to make a bad irresponsible choice, be mature, responsible and accountable to own it and to face the consequence that comes with it. Remember also, good choices come with good outcomes. Even Isaac Newton knew this when he showed the world using science that "to every action there is always an opposed equal reaction." You must also keep in mind that what you do to others will come back to you. Many call it karma but it is biblically written in Galatians 6:7 NIV "Do not be deceived: God cannot be mocked. **A man reaps what he sows.**"

> *"A life well lived is the best revenge."*
> *– Chloe Neill*

Even with knowing that God will get our revenge we must pay attention to our hearts. Our goal should not be that of a vengeful heart but a heart that doesn't rejoice when our enemy falls. (Proverbs 24:17) Yes, it is easier said than done.

As much as I want my husband and Ema's actions to catch up to them and to be revealed, which they most certainly will because I believe what God says in Proverbs 12:19 NLT ("Truthful words stand the test of time and lies will soon be exposed.") and in Luke 12:2 NIV, ("There is nothing concealed that will not be disclosed, or hidden that will not be made known.") I want more for my husband to turn back to God and to rekindle his relationship with God more than anything, because I know that's what God wants. There is much peace that comes with handing your antagonists over to God. When you let them go and release them and all that they have done to and against you, you are more able to forgive because you are trusting that God will deal with them and all they have done to you.

"Time is the most valuable thing a man can spend."
- Theophrastus

Every minute that passes in your life, you cannot get back. Don't waste you precious time, energy, and emotions on seeking revenge for the people who have wronged you. Do not give them that much power in your life, do not give them that much time of your life, and do not waste your emotions on the hurt they have caused you. What they did to you is done, it cannot be undone so let it go and trust God. Don't hang onto the hurt, bitterness, and anger; let it go and receive all of the good that God is offering you. When your hands are full, holding onto things that you do not need, your hands are unavailable to take what you deserve and need. Forgive the people who have hurt you so that God can move on your behalf.

"Always forgive your enemies; nothing annoys them so much."
– Oscar Wilde

Unforgiveness is a sin. Sin separates us from God. God cannot move on our behalf when we have unconfessed sin in our lives. God is so holy that he cannot be in the presence of sin let alone look at it. (Habakkuk 1:13) Before we ever knew Jesus, he died on a cross as the living sacrifice (1 Corinthians 15:3) on our behalf. Jesus didn't just willingly take on all of our sins and iniquities (Isaiah 53:5) but he became our sin (2 Corinthians 5:21) and in that moment God's presence was not there. Christ said himself while hanging on the cross, "My God, my God, why have you forsaken me?" (Matthew 27:46 NIV). Out of Christ's anguish from being separated from God, he cried out. Just like us, God can't be near us or help us when we have sin and unforgiveness in our lives. We must turn it over by professing it and asking God to help us. The anguish and pain that you feel from unforgiveness is stealing your peace, your joy, and your life.

"Repent then, and turn to God, so that your sins may be wiped out, that times of refreshing may come from the Lord."
Acts 3:19 (NASB)

Are you ready to forgive and take all of the goodness that comes from forgiving but you don't know how too? You don't know how to let go but you're tired of feeling the pain in your heart. You logically know that not forgiving is giving away your power but you can't seem to unclench your fists. You want your power back but the desire of unforgiveness is too strong?

"The weak can never forgive.
Forgiveness is the attribute of the strong."
- Mahatma Gandhi

I pose all of these questions to you because I know; I went through this process the hard way. It was so difficult for me to forgive Ema more than my husband. I could forgive my husband quickly because I loved him but I couldn't forgive Ema because she never stopped stealing from me or my children and she never apologized to me or my children and I am certain she never will. It was extremely difficult to release the unforgiveness in my heart for her; I knew that I needed to because most importantly that's what God wanted. I knew I needed to forgive because I was tired of it stealing my happiness and joy, I wanted to take my power back and not give the power to someone who was unworthy of it, but I knew more than anything that it was the unforgiveness that I held for Ema that was hindering my prayer life. God was not moving in my life and answering my prayers as quickly as he once was and I knew exactly why. I wanted God's favor back, I wanted answered prayers, I wanted to move forward into my destiny, and I wanted healing. But it was the unforgiveness I held onto that separated me from God. It took many prayers to get to the point that I could release Ema to God. I stood before God crying begging Him to help me release her. I asked God to forgive me for not forgiving. I begged God to help me release the unforgiveness, I didn't know how to so I asked Him to show me, and guess what, He did.

> *"To forgive is to set a prisoner free and*
> *discover that the prisoner was you."*
> *– Lewis B. Smedes*

The first thing you must do to release forgiveness is to set your mind to say, "I will forgive them, I want to forgive them" and then you pray. After you pray, you make your actions and your thoughts match your words. Your actions show God that you have faith in Him, and it is the combination of your faith and your prayers aligning with your actions that will move God's hand in your life.

I share this truth with you to empower you because it was when I finally figured out this combination, that I became unstoppable; because my relationship with God became unshakeable and so deep that nothing anyone said or did could stop God moving on my behalf because if God be for me, who can be against me? (Romans 8:31)

> *"It's what love does."*
> *– Bob Goff*

I can tell you honestly I did NOT want to forgive my husband or Ema at all. But because I loved God, I knew He wanted me to forgive them and so for that reason, it was my love for God that I chose to forgive them. I judiciously knew that everything I did not want to become would overtake me if I did not choose forgiveness. So I said, "I forgive my husband and I forgive Ema." I knew my feelings would catch up to my words soon or later, I just needed to keep saying it, especially in the moments I felt unforgiveness coming upon me. In layman terms, "Fake it 'til I make it." Or even better, as it's been said, "Faith it 'til you make it." The things that helped my feelings catch up to my words are the same things I am about to tell you to do in the next chapter. Let me help you pray to release forgiveness into your life. Pray this prayer:

Lord God Almighty,
I am in need of forgiveness for me and for others. My heart and my mind are in bondage to the unforgiveness I hold inside for _____ (put the name(s) of the person(s) you need to forgive). I want to release all of the misery, hurt, torment, bitterness, resentment, revenge, and pain that is consuming me. I want to give it to you and I want to take back my power and I want to be free. I want your peace, joy and happiness. I need help to forgive _____. I cannot do it alone. Help me to release them to you and in place give me all of the good that you want me to have from you. Your son died for me so

that I may be forgiven, your son died so I would be free, your son died so I could live a life filled with your abundance, help me to forgive. I forgive _____. I thank you Lord, for taking my unforgiveness I have for them from me and for setting me free. I thank you for the peace and sound mind you are giving me. I thank you that you love me enough to have your precious son die for me, and all of my sins and iniquities, though I am not worthy of such mercy and grace. I pray for _____ that your Holy Spirit may convict them and they too will turn to you. Thank you for hearing and answering my prayer. In Jesus' name. Amen.

"The best revenge is to not be like your enemies."
- Marcus Aurelius, Meditation

Chapter 5

PRAISE AND GRATITUDE

*"It is a good thing to give thanks unto the Lord, and
to sing praises unto thy name, O Most High."*
Psalm 92:1 (KJV)

Praise moves the hand of God. God loves to be worshipped. He created all things to sing His praises. Our existence alone is enough for Him to be worthy of our praises. When we praise God we not only give Him what is His and His alone but we are reminded of the many things He has done for us and our hearts become more grateful, our minds more understanding, our desires want more of Him and what He is and what He wants to give to us.

You are going through an extremely painful time in your life right now, though this may sound crazy it is very important that you PRAISE God through ALL of this. Trust me when I tell you, praise is an important key that opens the door to healing. Praise God that you are going through this right now because you are EXACTLY where you should be right now and the crazy part is, it is ALL for YOUR GROWTH, if you choose to grow from your circumstance.

When I was going through my separation, a very good Pastor friend told me to thank God for the things I was suffering from and experiencing. My response to him was, "Are you crazy? You are telling me to thank God that my husband left me and to be thankful for the pain that I am enduring?" My Pastor friend was right and this is what God showed me as I was going through it: God already knew that I was going to be left by the man I loved. God knew that I would be so hurt and devastated and that I would cry non-stop. God knew that I wanted death more than anything because the pain was so extreme. God knew my heart was so broken that I felt excruciating pain in the physical form throughout my body. He knew that I would lose sleep and that I would not eat and that I would fall into a depression. But God also knew, that I was strong enough to overcome, He knew that there was a fighter inside of me, though hidden at the time, that would keep propelling me forward. God also knew that I would become everything that He had created me to be. Having already known all this and watching, God also had a plan in store for me and for my life and He was ready to implement it as soon as I chose His way and not mine. It was so simple, all I had to do was choose; choose Him and then He would bottle up my tears, He would set me on a path to a life that was filled with love and joy, He would heal my broken heart, He would place the people I needed upon my path, He would test me, He would bless me and He would always make a way for me, especially when it was dark and I could see no way and God would let my heart feel real love for another again. God was already standing at the end with arms wide open just waiting for me to follow where He led, all I had to do was look up and say yes, I want and need You. All of that, all the things God had for me though I was not deserving, was and is worthy of my praises for Him.

Once I looked up and I decided that I wanted happiness, that I wanted joy, that I wanted peace, and that I was willing to do whatever it took to get there; I chose God. I followed Him and I praised Him. He not only led me closer to Himself, but closer to my destiny, closer to a life greater than I could ever imagine, but more importantly, He made me more like Jesus. It was the overwhelming pain that God allowed me to endure that led me to the choice to cry out for Him, desiring to be as far away from all of my pain, and this desire led me to my choice that led me to my transformation. It was through my pain, that God transformed me physically, mentally, emotionally, and spiritually. It was through my praises for God that helped motivate, if you will, His hand. My praises for God, proved to Him that I trusted Him with all that I had left: my life, my future, and my heart.

Believe me, I know it is very hard right now for you to find things to thank God for but if you start with the little things, you will start to see bigger things. I give you my word, if you start to praise God now, you will see that He will give you greater things to praise Him for and you will feel unworthy because you won't be able to fathom how a God so majestic and powerful could love you and give you things that you don't deserve. I know, because I felt this. I was so thankful because I really did not deserve the things He gave me and yet He continues to bless me. Through my praises, He created in me a heart of gratitude. God is a God who keeps His promises, when you choose Him, when you praise Him, He will do everything in His power that is for your best interest to help you fulfill your purpose in this life.

Here are a few examples to help you get started, say these repetitiously and watch how your heart changes, how your perspective on all things become clearer, how life will feel and seem so simple and how you will have a sense of peace that is beyond your understanding. Remember, **praise leads to gratitude, gratitude leads to peace, peace leads to freedom, and freedom leads to happiness.**

Examples: I praise you God because you are majestic and victorious. I thank you for all that I am going through. Though I do not understand I know that you do. I am thankful for today, another day you have given me. I thank you that you have already gone before me and have made a way through every situation I will encounter. I thank you for the blessings you have bestowed upon me and for the people you have placed upon my path to help me. You are the King of Kings and all glory and honor belongs to you. You're the only God that reigns and the God above all gods, yet you love me more than I know. You are beautiful and you made all things good, you created me in your image so I am beautiful, I am victorious. I praise you and I give thanks for your holiness, mercy, and grace because you extend all of these to me. You are worthy of my praises. All power is yours because you are the I Am. You are love and you love me. I worship you because you love me, thank you for loving me. I exalt your name above all names because you are good and glorious. You are majestic and all majesty is yours and yours alone. Blessed be your name. You are the only maker and creator of all, you create a way for me all of the time. All things I have are because of you. I praise Your Son, Jesus Christ because your design is like no other. I thank and glorify you oh God because you cause my feet not to slip. Let all that is in me bless you Lord and let all praises of mine belong to you alone. Father God you are my provider, you give me food to eat, drink to drink and you give me a place to rest my head. High praises to the Lord of lords and King of kings because you bring me people to help me and to bless me. My heart desires you and you alone. Gracious and merciful are thee, you're the King of glory. Thank you for the sun that shines upon my face. Thank you for the wind that cools my body. I am thankful for eyes to see the beauty that surrounds me. My ears hear the joyful noises that encompasses me. My heart is thankful for all things good that are to come to me. I look forward to the future because it is bright, it is peaceful, and it is whole. (See more examples at the end of this chapter.)

When you begin to fear or doubt, open your mouth and speak things that you are thankful for out loud; even for the smallest most ordinary things. If you cannot find things to be thankful for just say these three simple words, "Thank You God." When you are down read the following scripture out loud and pay attention to your mood and how you feel when you are done.

Psalm 145 (KJV)
"I exalt you, my God the King; and praise
your name forever and ever.
I will praise you every day; I will honor
your name forever and ever.
Yahweh is great and is highly praised; His
greatness is unsearchable.
One generation will declare your works to the
next and will proclaim your mighty acts.
I will speak of your splendor and glorious
majesty and your wonderful works.
They will proclaim the power of your awe-inspiring
acts, and I will declare your greatness. They will give
a testimony of your great goodness and will joyfully
sing of your righteousness. The Lord is gracious and
compassionate, slow to anger and great in faithful love.
The Lord is good to everyone; His compassion
rests on all He has made.
All You have made will thank You, Lord; the godly will
praise You. They will speak of the glory of Your kingdom and
will declare Your might, informing all people of Your
mighty acts and of the glorious splendor of Your kingdom.
Your kingdom is an everlasting kingdom; Your rule is for
all generations. The Lord is faithful in all His words and
gracious in all His actions. The Lord helps all who fall; He
raises up all who are oppressed. All eyes look to you, and
you give them their food at the proper time. You open your
hand and satisfy the desire of every living thing. The Lord
is righteous in all His ways and gracious in all His acts.
The Lord is near all who call out to Him, all who call out
to Him with integrity. He fulfills the desires of those who

fear Him; He hears their cry for help and saves them. The
Lord guards all those who love Him, but He destroys all
the wicked. My mouth will declare Yahweh's praise; let
every living thing praise His holy name forever and ever."

"When you are grateful, fear disappears,
and abundance appears."
– Anthony Robbins

Remember that you must choose to always think positive and
loving things not only about yourself but also about your life.
You must seek daily to find the good in EVERY situation. You
actively look for and at the beauty and majesty that surrounds
you each and every day. Sit quietly and just listen to your breath
and in that moment thank God for giving you that breath of life
and then thank Him more for the many other good things in your
life. When you feel like you have not forgiven your foe, speak out
loud, "I have already forgiven them." You must read your Bible to
learn what God wants to tell you and the most important thing
is to be thankful for everything that is in your life both good and
even the bad.

Be thankful that God has your best interest at heart and
He is allowing you to go through the bad so that you come out
more positive and stronger. Your bad moments not only teach
you a lesson but it will help you to grow as a person in character,
experience, thought, and in life. You will look back one day on all
of this and say, "Wow, I AM thankful that I went through that."
And you will realize it was all to make you into the person you
will become.

If you don't know or have forgotten what God promises you,
I have included a list of His promises for you at the end of the
book. When you don't know what to speak, read them out loud
and mediate on them until you come to a place that you believe
it and you know that God will keep those promises to you. I can

tell you from my experience, God ALWAYS keeps His promise to those who love Him. He kept every single one of His promises to me and He can and will do it for you if you follow the things I am teaching you. Remember, God gives you free will to choose. **How you choose will determine the path you will travel in life.**

Here are a few more examples of things to be thankful for and blanks for you to fill in for other things you are thankful for.

Thank You Lord for:

- my job.	- my family.	- my friends.	- the seasons.	- my sight.	- my ability to hear.
-my home.	- the view.	- my clothes.	- the food I eat.	- my vehicle.	- my children.
- the shoes on my feet.		- the air I breathe.	- my health.	- my ability to walk.	– my pets.

_____   _____   _____   _____   _____

_____   _____   _____   _____   _____

_____   _____   _____   _____   _____

Chapter 6

TRUST

*"Trust in the Lord with all your heart; and lean not on
your own understanding. In all your ways acknowledge
Him and He will make your paths straight."*
Proverbs 3:5-6 (AMP)

Trust is one of the hardest things to do. By nature we often want to always be in control. To trust someone is scary, it makes you vulnerable, maybe even left to feel naïve. Trust however is an important fundamental foundational part of every relationship.

I look back now at my divorce and I can see with understanding and clarity as to why God allowed my husband to walk away from me. It was not easy, and my heart was sad but my husband's calamitous choices while we were married was deteriorating who I was as well as killing my spirit. Of the two evils, the divorce was lesser of the two. My husband in his free will chose to walk in the opposite direction of me, downward and I was never meant to walk that dire path. That was not the path that would lead me into my destiny. I was growing in my relationship with God, I was ready to advance to the next level in my life, and I was choosing to continually work on becoming a better person each day. My husband however, was not; he was stuck and as I watched him move in the opposite direction of me doing the things that were not good for him, for me, or our family, I could not on my own bisect us. Remember, I had unknowingly lost my identity in him. I also didn't want my family destroyed and as exhausting and excruciating as it was at times, begging him to do right by us and for his own sake, I kept fighting for our marriage the best I knew how at the time. God allowed it because my husband would keep me stuck and keep me from fulfilling my destiny and fulfilling God's will and purpose for my life not to mention, God allows us to use our free will.

Like an eagle, I am extremely loyal and I was willing to keep trying to fight for my marriage so God allowed <u>him</u>, my husband, to walk away from <u>me</u> because I wasn't going to quit. It was exceptionally hard to let him go and it took much time to do so because I adored him and the love I had for him was like no other I had for anyone else, my love for him ran deep and I loved him with every part of me though he may not have been able to see it or feel it because my actions and reactions came from a hurting, desperate, bleeding heart.

God knew that I would survive but He also knew what choices I would make and He knew that the cutting away of our marriage from my life, as much as He hated it (Malachi 2:16), was going to make me stronger and better but, He also knew that I would trust Him and trust that He would see me through to the end, not leaving me alone and that He would transform me in a way that nothing else could. I can honestly say that through the process of me letting go I could literally feel half of who I was and half of my heart be torn apart. It was the single hardest thing I've ever had to do but it was also the very thing that made me stronger and literally made me fearless but it more importantly caused me to trust God completely.

* * * * * * * * * * * * * * * * * * *

The things that happened to me during my childhood created insecurity within me that caused me to not be very trusting of people, especially of men. Then going into my marriage, my husband who delighted in the attention from others, especially the attention from women fed that insecurity often only to prove in the latter part of our marriage that my insecurity was real. Feeling insecure and not very trusting of people is a shackle that kept me and keeps many people in bondage. It wasn't until I lost absolutely everything in my life that I finally had the opportunity to learn trust. I had to lose my marriage, my homes, my truck, my money, my family, and my identity in order for me to learn to trust. I had nothing literally, let me restate that, by the grace of God, I still had my children and I was thankful for it.

Having to care for my children with nothing was very scary. To know that other lives are dependent on you is, not only a huge responsibility but also a serious one and it brings with it an overwhelming sense of fear. It was when I had nothing but God to turn to that I learned what trust was and what trusting someone was really about. It was also when I learned that there was one person I could count on no matter what, who would never let me down. ALL of my friends and family; have let me down at one time or another, just as I am certain I have probably done the same to them.

When God says in the Bible, "For the word of the Lord is right and true; he is faithful in all he does." (Psalm 33:4 NIV), He was not lying. I'm a walking living testimony of that truth. When I had no food, God brought me food, when I had no place to live, He housed me, when I wanted to compete in a body building competition, He brought me a pro body builder to train me, when I lost my vehicle, He provided another, when I had no money, He supplied my needs etc. EVERY time I needed something God provided. When I had nobody, He was there.

To this day, I still don't trust people one hundred percent but I don't need to because I have God. I am sure it is partially a protective mechanism that I have created within myself because I am weary from coming from a place of many broken promises; having so many people tell me they will do something and then they don't follow through or they don't keep their word.

A person who keeps their word, I have much respect for. My reason for this is; at the end of our life or when we are at rock bottom, when we have nothing else, the only thing we are left with is our word and our character. How well a person can keep their word is a measure of how much character they have and it is the measure that I measure others. I am one who keeps her word, I won't make promises that I can't keep or never planned on keeping. It drives me insane when someone says they are going to do something for me or with me and they never do, and when the time comes, the truth reveals that the only reason they ever said they would do what they had promised was either to impress me, to win points with me, to get their way or because they were to cowardly to state what was true in their heart. In the end, they did neither; they didn't win any points with me, if anything they ended up losing some of my respect for them. I have had to let the expectation go for many people I care about who said they would be there or that they would come through for me. Choosing to do this has alleviated much undue stress and frustration from my life. It still irks me somewhat because I want people to be people of their word, but so many people, unfortunately cannot. This is not to say, that you shouldn't trust people, I am not saying that at all. There are red flags that will show you when a person is completely untrustworthy; I am speaking in terms of overall. Life is so much simpler when we don't put all of our trust in people or expect them to always be there, to always be understanding, to always be supportive, to always be on your side, to always be encouraging, etc. No human being has the ability to be everything you need or need to trust, this I have come to learn. If you can come to a place where you can accept that very fact, your life too will be much easier and you won't face as many disappointments.

Though many people have a difficult time being trustworthy or people of their word, I want to encourage you to be a trustworthy person as well as keeping your word always, despite how others are towards you.

Why not try, if you haven't already, place your trust in God and see what He can and will do for you.

The best proof of love is trust."
- Joyce Brothers

Chapter 7

ACTION

"Action is the foundational key to all success."
- Pablo Picasso

Action is a word that entails movement, activity, and motion. Action is not inert and never remains idle. In order for change to occur, an action must be set into motion.

DECIDE → COMMIT → ACT

It took some time for me to get to the point of taking action. I want you to know that as soon as I was discarded by my husband I didn't immediately say, "Okay enough is enough." I wasn't that strong at the time and I honestly was exhausted by the time he decided to walk away. I had fought so hard trying to do everything in my power to save my marriage and to keep my family in tact but it all seemed so futile. I was the only one trying to keep the promise we had made to each other over eighteen years prior though he was not. I fell into a depression and I knew that I needed to get off of the couch and change my scenery before I became completely paralyzed to the despair that consumed me. I knew that I needed to be more than that for my children and though it was harmful for me and would inevitably lead to my ruin, I knew that if something didn't change, the emotional state I was in would chiefly begin the expeditious rate of speed towards the deterioration of my children's outcome. They were already dealing with the consequences of their father's recklessness and they did not need me to add to their emotional torment. This desire to do more for them and to be more for them caused me to get off of the couch that I sulked on day after day and to get out of my pajamas and into the gym.

On this morning, I decided to get dressed into workout clothes while my children got ready for school. My normal routine was to wake them up for school and let them get themselves ready for school while I moved from my bed to the couch where I would lay waiting for them to tell me that they were ready to go to school. Then I would get off of the couch in my pajamas and drive them to school and then returned home to lie on the couch until it was time to pick them up. This day was different, this day I made a choice, I decided to do better to become better to take control of my life and no longer be a victim. After dropping my children off at school I drove straight to the gym so that I would not be tempted to fall back into my depressing routine. As I walked into the gym, I did not know what I was going to do so I went straight to a treadmill and hit the quick start button. As the belt on the treadmill began to turn, I took my first step. The first step, a step I did not know then, was the first step that led to my transformational change, the first step that took me from victim to victorious and the first step towards my healing.

It was on the treadmill that I would walk and think; finding myself talking with God. First, bombarding Him with questions of why and then walking, if you will, into a closer relationship with Him. It was during my times in prayer with God that He helped me move from talking about my circumstance to taking action. Actions that would not only change and reset the course path that led to my destiny, my purpose for which I was created.

The following 10 steps I am about to share with you, were the very steps that God took me through to get me to where I am right now. Many of them were extremely hard, not just mentally, but emotionally and even physically. I say physically because emotional pain can be felt physically as well. God literally transformed me from the inside out. When He was done taking me through the valley of the shadow of death and keeping me in the desert, ironically, He literally placed me physically in the desert to live, He created a new person in me. He made me stronger physically, mentally, and emotionally, He made me more confident, more faithful and trusting of Him and He set me on a foundation that was unshakeable. He taught me whom I was and that I was His, to the point where the opinions of others no longer affected me and could no longer affect me. God helped me take back my power and taught me how to never release it to another person again. He made me strong, confident, bold, and immovable, in essence, unstoppable.

"Set your mind on things above, not on earthly things."
Colossians 3:2 (NIV)

1. SET YOUR MIND

The first action you must make after choosing victory is to make up your mind, to set your mind. The Bible states clearly to set your mind, that is not an option, rather, it is a command. You choose your thoughts; nobody else can do this for you. You must decide for yourself, "I am not going to allow this situation or person(s) to affect me or steal my happiness. I am not going to waste my time thinking thoughts that are no good for me that do nothing but steal my time and joy. Enough is enough! This person(s) does not deserve this much power in my life." Once you choose to reclaim your power over your own life, you must then commit to the work required to become victorious. Stop mentally replaying the hurt done to you and reset your mind on seeking out a new way to get to your goals.

> *"...but I focus on this one thing: Forgetting the past*
> *and looking forward to what lies ahead,"*
> Philippians 3:13 (NLT)

2. COMMIT

Commitment requires action. Your actions must reinforce your choice, your decision to be victorious. One way to put your choice into action is by choosing <u>not</u> to speak your feelings that derive from fear or hurt. Hurt and fear are always the underlying emotions that usually always leads to anger, insecurities, doubt, and misled reasoning -- all resulting in the destruction of your heart, your peace, your mind, even your sleep, but more importantly your life. Commitment is not always easy and it always entails a plan and requires work. Commitment means to keep doing what you have pledged to do even when you don't feel like doing it anymore. Commitment is keeping a promise you made whether it is to yourself or to another person. Commitment is when you keep trying even after failing. **Commitment assuredly always leads to success. To be successful, your commitment must be absolute.**

> *"Think on things that are true, noble, right, pure,*
> *lovely, admirable, excellent or praise worthy."*
> Philippians 4:8 (KJV)

3. GUARD YOUR THOUGHTS

Once you set your mind and you are committed, you must guard your thoughts. Guarding your thoughts is not an easy task; it's a skill that takes practice. When an unkind, judgmental, or negative thought enters your mind, STOP IT IMMEDIATELY do not allow it to continue. Do not allow it to develop into something worse or more damaging. Change your thoughts instantly and start thinking about something else. If you are having an unfavorable or negative thought about someone or an incident, stop thinking on that thought, instead, change your thought and remember something good about the person or try to find something you can take from it to learn and to grow. This is not to say you shouldn't examine the matter but try to do it from a rational point of view, where you disconnect your emotions from the facts so that you can figure out what the underlying issue(s) is.

You should not waste your time meditating on your misfortunes. If you have a difficult time changing your thoughts, I suggest maybe trying one of these alternatives: look around you and begin to people watch, stop and take notice to the wind blowing through the trees, pay attention to your breath, turn on uplifting music and sing and or dance, or go watch a movie, preferably a comedy, go play a sport, do a craft, or read a book.

A good man/woman brings good things stored up in his/her heart, and an evil man/woman brings evil things stored up in his/her heart. For the mouth speaks what the heart is full of."
Luke 6:45 (NIV)

4. LOOK INWARD

Spend time alone and think about the things you feel, the things you have gone through, your experiences, listen to the words that come out of your mouth, and then decide which of those things you do not like and want or need to change about yourself, to change for the better. Get rid of the things in your life that are holding you down, the things that are keeping you from moving forward, and remove the people in your life who are toxic to you and your goal of victory. Once you look inward, take accountability and responsibility for your shortcomings and your misdeeds without making excuses for them, then forgive yourself, let it go and give it to God because you cannot change what has already happened then begin to do things that help you to change towards becoming a better you.

> *"Each of you must take responsibility for doing the*
> *creative best you can with your own life."*
> *Galatians 6:5 (AMP)*

5. TAKE RESPONSIBILITY AND ACCOUNTABILITY

I became free and I took back my power when I chose to let my pride go and to accept responsibility for my actions and my part in the break down of my marriage. Yes, ultimately our marriage ended as a result of my husband's selfish choice to break apart our family and to walk away but I did contribute as well throughout the marriage as I shared in a previous chapter. It always takes two to either build up or tear down a relationship. It were the little foxes that I described to you previously that you must be mindful of in all of your relationships. It is these little foxes—situations and discordances that will slowly and microscopically eat away at the outcome that we want or expect if they continue to go unnoticed and unresolved. Often times we write them off as trivial instances and we discount them as being diminutive moments but we don't realize their long-term effects if we allow them to keep occurring.

No matter how embarrassing, shameful or guilty you feel about your misdeeds you must acknowledge them. Take responsibility and accountability for them. With a sincere heart, apologize. Commit to making it better, to make a wrong right, and to move forward never to repeat your misdeed(s).

> *"Get rid of all bitterness, rage and anger, brawling*
> *and slander, along with every form of malice. Be*
> *kind and compassionate to one another, forgiving*
> *each other, just as in Christ God forgave you."*
> *Ephesians 4:31-32 (NIV)*

6. FORGIVE

Forgiveness is very important and an essential part of healing. It will be hard at first to forgive but set your mind on forgiving the one(s) who hurt you. Say it, even if you don't feel it. Ask God to help you forgive the person(s) that hurt you. When they do something or say something that hurts you, say to yourself, "I forgive them." I promise, soon your feelings will catch up to your words. Forgiveness is a vital step towards freedom and with it comes empowerment. If you do anything, make forgiveness your ultimate goal. Forgiveness is a choice; choose it, not for them but for your sake.

"The tongue has the power of life and death,
and those who love it will eat its fruit."
Proverbs 18:21 (NIV)

7. SPEAK LIFE

Every time you have an adverse thought enter your mind and or when you open your mouth to speak, be conscious of the words that are about to leave your lips. The words you speak hold power; they can either build up or tear down. When you have a problem, do not dwell on it rather, meditate on (Joshua 1:8) encouraging words (see Speaking Gods Promises and Bible Verses section) instead of talking about your problem(s) find positive things to say. This doesn't just remove negative thoughts from your mind but it will leave you feeling better and happier about your situation and life. It will also teach you how to look at things in a different light. If somebody says something to demean you or tear you down you say out loud to him or her, "I am sorry you feel that way but I am not _____." You fill the blank in with the word(s) they used. After you rebuke the words spoken to you or over you, you reinforce your thoughts with positive words spoken out loud, for example, "I am a child of the most high God. I am a good person. I am _____. " Etc. Fill in the blank with positive and affirming truths about yourself. (See Speak Life section and in the workout to find truths to speak) If someone speaks against your dreams speak positive statements that go against what they spoke and remind yourself that you WILL one day live your dream; "I will become a great published writer watch and see!"

If the person who has hurt you is speaking lies about you. Do not choose to respond in the same manner, no matter how bad it hurts. If you speak the words caused from hurt, you will end up being more hurt and your heart will begin to harden and you will not be able to free yourself from the bondage that comes from listening to corrupt and destructive words. For example, If I were to say repeatedly, "I hate my husband for what he did to me" my feelings would rehash the pain that came from the lies, the betrayal, the lack of loyalty, and the unwillingness on his part to fight for our relationship etc. and the more I repeat the words, "I hate" I train myself and my mind to think that I do hate and the more I hear it the more it resonates in my head until I begin to believe it. Once I believe that I hate him, the hate then drops down into my heart and then I become everything that particularizes hate (misery, demoralization, anger, unkindness, envy, revenge, resentment, hostility etc.). Once the feeling of hate resonates in my heart, my actions, my thoughts, and my words begin to engulf my life. If I were to allow hate to enter my heart, it would begin to harden my heart, preventing love from flowing into it and more importantly flowing out of it. Having hate in my heart and speaking the words "I hate" (or any other ruinous word(s)) would only continue to refuel and empower the loathing that I already felt and it would commence the genesis of who I would become (For as he or she thinketh in his or her heart, so is he or she. (Proverbs 23:7)), and the more I hate the more it steals from me, stealing my joy, my peace, my sleep, my time and my life. One thing to remember, the truth always comes to light, so any lies that are spoken about you will soon or later be found as a lie and the liar will then be known as a liar.

"Death and life are in the power of the tongue."
Proverbs 18:21 (ESV)

The mistreatment by others should not lead you to inflict masochistic delirium upon yourself, leading to the wallowing in your own misery like victims often do. This self-destructive state will also cause you to do things that are unkind and ungodly, like gossip and slander etc.

Distance yourself or break off unhealthy relationships with people who gossip, speak untruths, or who always seem to have a negative thing to say about anything, everyone, and everything etc. You must choose to only listen to truth and not gossip and you do not participate in gossip or negative judgmental conversation about others, especially the person who may have hurt you. Nothing good ever comes from gossip.

Besides segregating yourself from toxic people who spew toxicity from their lips you must also choose to speak affirmative words about yourself, and you must also only listen to things that build you up. Whether they are sermons, encouraging music, (see song list at the end of the book) or motivational speakers etc. Watch movies or television shows that will encourage you or make you laugh. Read books that will teach you or inspire you.

"The righteous must choose their friends carefully,
for the way of the wicked leads them astray."
Proverbs 12:26 (ESV)

8. CHOOSE YOUR FRIENDS CAREFULLY

Who you choose to spend your time with will immensely impact the type of life you live as well as the path you take and more importantly determine whether or not you step into your destiny. When you choose to be a child of God, God places people on your path to help you, encourage you, inspire you, challenge you, and to help you grow for the better. Whether you are a child of God or not, **who you choose to spend your time with will determine the type of life you will lead**. If you are spending time with people who are not good for you, you will not and cannot meet the right people who are good for you; the people who will help you get to higher ground as well as new opportunities. You must make a conscious choice to surround yourself with people who sincerely have your best interest at heart, who will encourage you, and who will be lovingly honest with you even if it hurts.

It's not too problematic to understand, good people and bad people just do not associate with one another, everything about them just don't equal to the other, metaphorically they're like chickens and eagles. Chickens represent people who are lazy, critical, disrespectful, indifferent, people who would cause you to compromise who you are; your beliefs, your morals, your ethics, and or your standards, people whom gossip, who bring you down and talk down to you, and are mediocre people who drain your energy. Chickens are people who are stuck exactly where they are and they don't move forward in careers, in relationships, or in life.

When you are stuck you cannot to move forward, you cannot advance, you cannot grow or change, and you are unable to move into your destiny. You become like the type of people you continually choose to hang out with — the chickens.

Eagles represent people of excellence: they're successful, considerate, honorable, kind, generous, committed, motivated and focused. They are people of action. Their positive and encouraging characteristics, if you spend time with them, will rub off onto you. In Proverbs 13:20 (NASB) it says, "If you "walk with wise men you become wise" and in Proverbs 22:24 (NLT), "Do not become friends with angry people or be associated with them or you will become like them."

> *"Become wise by walking with the wise; hangout*
> *with fools and watch your life fall to pieces."*
> *Proverbs 13:20 (NASB)*

I mention chicken and eagles because I was on the Internet watching the live feed of an eagle's nest. It showed the mother and father eagle as they prepared the arrival of their baby eagles. It made me wonder what kind of life they had so I began to research it to read and to learn more. I was fascinated with what I learned, and what is more amazing is God speaks of the characteristics of an eagle in the Bible. Interestingly the characteristics of an eagle in the Bible are the exact characteristics the eagle really possesses. Let's look at the characteristics of an eagle compared to that of a chicken.

Chickens spend their days scratching the ground and walking around their coops; slow, relaxed with no sense of urgency or purpose with their chests puffed out strutting their heads back and forth, they act as if they are somebody important but in reality they're only a "somebody" in their own chicken coop. The minute a person or an animal comes into their coop or chases after them they run fast cackling and clucking loudly. Chickens though they have wings, never get off the ground, they flap their wings but they get nowhere. Chickens don't travel any further than they're fenced in area permits but when you watch them, they never really try to fly to get out of their coop (situation) and they only associate with one another and on some occasion maybe with a duck, or pigeon. When a storm arises the first thing they do is to run as fast as they can clucking and flapping all the way to the coop to huddle with all of the other chickens.

Eagles are the extreme opposite of a chicken. They build their nests in the highest rock and don't mind being alone (independent). When they decide to commit to another eagle, they are committed until death. Eagles don't mind being uncomfortable and are always willing to step outside of their comfort zone to accomplish the task at hand. Eagles are brave. When an eagle sees a storm (problem) it will wait for it then fiercely enter it head on using the thermal currents from the storm to raise them higher above the storm. Eagles are also very focused; they will lock their sights onto a goal, their prey for example, and they will study it and outsmart it in order to conquer it. Eagles are patient. Eagles take time every day to rejuvenate. When an eagle begins to get worn down and aren't as efficient as they need to be, they will take time to revitalize themselves, sharpening again their talons, plucking out their feathers one by one so new ones can grow back in. Eagles will endure the pain of pulling all of their feathers out in order to remove all parasites and dirt from their body (lives) in order to be better equipped so that they can continue with their purpose. Though it takes 40 days for an eagle's new feathers to grow back in, they don't concern themselves with the pain or the length of the process they're more concerned about their progress. When you look at an eagle you witness strength, beauty, might, courage, fearlessness, determination and confidence. Eagles are usually seen flying alone, sometimes you will see a few of them together either soaring or perched up high on a tree. This is because eagles keep their inner circle small and elite, they only associate with other eagles that have the same characteristics (interests/goals), not to mention, they don't have the inclination to waste their time with other birds that do not have similar goals.

Birds of a feather flock together, chickens cluck with chickens (symbolize people who are stuck) and eagles only soar with eagles (symbolize people of excellence). You can only rise as high as the people who are in your life. As I do often, at least every few months, I will re-evaluate my friends or the people I associate with. If I don't feel a person is "good" for me, meaning, they bring me down, they're always negative and critical, they always make excuses, they don't keep their word, they lie, are untrustworthy, they gossip, are disrespectful, or they try to take advantage and use others to get ahead in some way shape or form I will either cut myself off completely from them or I will begin to distance myself from them. We get one life, that means we only get one shot at it and we can not get back the time we waste or lose and our time here upon this earth is short and can end at any moment. Why waste this succinct time with people who do not compliment your life in a positive and productive way? I choose to remove people from my life, including family, that do not help me serve my purpose or have the same values as I do. If you want to know where you will be in a few years, take a good look at your friends. Are they like chickens or like eagles?

People are in our lives for a season, they come and they go. Each person in our life was placed on our path to help us in some way shape or form during our journey upon this earth, just as we are in their lives: to serve a purpose for them. The people in our lives are their to either teach us a lesson, to help us get to the next level in our life, or to help us grow whether in spirit or in character. Now you must make a choice, will you spend your time with chickens or with eagles?

> *"Therefore, be careful how you walk, not as an unwise man but as wise, making the most of your time..."*
> *Ephesians 5:15-16 (NASB)*

9. SPEND YOUR TIME WISELY

How you spend your time is an essential element in moving from a broken place to an empowered victorious place. The way you spend your time should reflect your choices and your commitment towards change and the reconfirming of your desire for healing of your heart.

Spend your time doing something that will better you. Put your energy into finding other ways to get to your productive positive goals. Use the hurt you feel to fuel and drive you towards your goals and towards where you envision yourself. Revisit your gifts and talents and share them. Know that your gifts and talents that you have were not given to you from God to keep to yourself but for you to give to others. Why not share your God given gift with the world, more likely than not, the world, if not someone needs to be blessed by it. Remember, **everything in life has a purpose that is bigger than you.**

> *"Living with intention means saying no to the*
> *things that aren't important to us so we can*
> *say yes to what matters most."*
> – Crystal Paine

10. LIVE INTENTIONALLY

To live intentionally means to live on purpose. To do things with intent. Each day you must wake up and choose to be glad that you are alive, thankful that you were given another day, another chance, another opportunity, etc. The values and core beliefs that you have should be used as your moral compass and the standard you set each day for yourself. If you follow and adhere to the standards that you hold, you will live with a clear conscience and you will be more apt to listen to your own inner voice rather than the cackling of others who may not share the same level of beliefs. **Never lower your standards for anyone, rather, let others rise to meet them.** You must set your priorities in life. Take a look at what and who is important to you, once you do that, make time and effort to do those things and to spend your valuable time with those people who at the end of the day matter to you most. Do what you are most passionate about, when you are passionate about something it brings you joy, it makes sense, and it is fulfilling. Use your passions to make a difference in the life of another person. You were blessed with a gift so that you could bless somebody else. Be always thankful with a heart and mind filled with gratitude. Remember that everything we have does not belong to us. We arrived into the world naked and with nothing and when we die we cannot bring anything with us. Everything we have is borrowed, even the very air we breathe, we must return it with every exhale. **Be in the moment.** Being in the moment means to be present, to be aware, to appreciate exactly where you are and who you are with at any given time. Cherish every moment and do your best to live with no regret because you never know when your life may end. Go do something that is not only advantageous but also adventurous.

God created you to do amazing things and to enjoy: his mountains, his oceans, his skies, his beaches, and his lakes, his everything. Go do something with them. Climb to the top of a hill or mountain and just sit there and take in the picturesque view, lay under a tree and watch and listen to the wind rustle through the leaves, sit on a beach and watch the waves flow in and out, go to a park and watch the birds fly and socialize with one another, take a hike through a national park and feel the air as it touches your face or just sit alone and listen to your own breath. Do things that will not only better your soul but your life. Take a class in something you would like to either get better at or always wanted to learn. Take up a new language or art (dance, music, painting, etc.). Join a bible study group, volunteer at church or at a shelter, help support a cause. Go to a ballet or a musical. Go do things that will surround you with like-minded people and things that will take you away and your mind off of your situation. It won't only keep your mind occupied but when you get through the storm you will come out a little bit better than when you went into it. Purposefully go and become a better you.

**Be genuine. Live purposefully. Live authentic.
Live intentionally. Be intentional.**

Chapter 8

REDEMPTIVE LOVE

As I reflect back, I can say without a doubt that this season of my life was *the* very worst of my entire life. Humorously enough, it simultaneously was also the very best part of it. With all that has happened to me, looking back now, it seems as if it played on fast-forward though during the most trying times it moved at a glacial speed.

I can remember vividly back to the New Years Eve, that in hindsight was a pivotal moment that catapulted me to where I am today, recalling the expectation and excitement that filled every part of my body as I waited anxiously for the clock to strike midnight, ready to devour all that the New Year had in store for me. I was ready for change, ready for a new beginning, I was prepared to end the old and commence with all that was new. Little did I know that everything that I wanted, I would get, just not in the manner I anticipated and hoped for.

Instead, the new year was extensively filled with grief, endless pain and hurt, trial after trial, test after test, betrayal after betrayal, loss after loss; there was more negative and sad moments than there were happy ones for me. I lost everything in one year, having lost: the relationship and friendship of my best friend, my "soul mate" who was my husband, my marriage, my family being torn apart, my identity, my self esteem, "friends", my job as a Marine

Corps wife, and my financial stability; which sent me into financial ruin not by my choice. I no longer had the material things that I once took pride in, the things I had worked so hard to achieve, to attain, the markers to which identified my "successes"; my eight houses, my two boats, all of my cars, my toys, my credit score, my saving accounts, my money markets, the ability to vacation twice a year etc. My entire fortune and empire ceased to exist. I went from living on the golf course to living in a RV trailer to literally being homeless for a couple of months. There was a period where I did not have enough money to feed my children, so I went hungry. My only form of transportation broke down and then the means to which it was to be fixed was stolen, however, it was totaled in an accident shortly after and I did not have enough insurance coverage to replace it; resulting in the complete loss of that as well. I believe I experienced the most betrayal a person could possibly endure by so many people in a short amount of time, I am astonished looking back, that I was able to keep going with all of the "knife wounds" I had received in my back. The family and "friends" that I was certain would be there for me in my time of need, was not, I had been abandoned by them too. These were only a few of the many atrocities that I endured that year. My entire life as I knew it ended, my world had come crashing down. Everything that I thought was true about my life turned out to be a fabrication of my imagination.

Anyone who has endured a deep heartache can relate to the stabbing pain that consumes your heart at such a devastating loss.

As I am left to reason over ALL that I lost; the things I fought so hard to keep, the things that were stolen from me, the relationships that were torn from my life and the things I thought were the foundation to my existence, I sit here and I write, tears falling from my eyes, with a smile upon my face and a heart full of joy and thankfulness for the loss of it all.

For those of you who can not believe or understand why my wounded heart rejoices or how I am able to be thankful after having gone through so much agony, I can only sum it up in one word, God. Like I stated previously, this is not a "religious" story, but rather the redemptive love story of a woman who despite all of her shortcomings, failures, and disappointments is still standing by the undeserving grace and mercy of God, a God who chose her when nobody else did, who fought for her when nobody else would, and who loved her when she felt unlovable. This particular chapter of my life is just part of my testimony.

My entire life, I "knew" God, I did what every "Christian" was suppose to do: I went to church on Sunday and I even brought my Bible with me, I was nice to people, I gave to the needy, donated to good causes, I volunteered when I could, I helped my friends and strangers, I said my prayers before I went to bed, I "gave" my life to Jesus, and so on; I did everything that a textbook Christian was suppose to do. I lived a "safe" Christian life. But then...there's always a but...but then, as the clock struck midnight on that New Years Eve, the genesis of everything I asked for began it's fruition into existence...and so the summation of my year began...

Through all of my pain and heartache, through all that I endured, during my moments of abandonment, in my time of confusion and frustration, in my rages of hate, anger, bitterness, in my loneliness, in my periods of complete utter fear with no signs of hope, and through my darkest moments when I coveted death more than anything...God showed Himself not only <u>real</u> and <u>true</u> but <u>faithful</u>.

God had literally placed me in the desert in every sense of the word, to include the physical (God had moved our family to the desert in California). He planted me dead center in the sweltering heat, in the insufferable dryness, and in the scarcity of many things, in every aspect of my life. It was in the "desert" when the comprehension of what I did not want, the ending of my eighteen-year marriage, was quickly becoming my reality. I fought as hard as I could to keep it but I lost and I lost everything along with it. As my three children and I literally watch the man that was suppose to fight for us walk out the front door and walk away from us, a fighter and a defender slowly and subtly began to rise up within me, though at that very moment I did not know the level to which she existed or when she would even show up.

Days and weeks began to pass and I fell into a depression. I could not understand how my life went from us being the "poster family for Gap" to complete turmoil and disarray leaving me with no identity or self worth, not even knowing who I was let alone what I liked or wanted—the collateral damage from the break-up was too much. I was exhausted, I was despondent, I was useless, and I was fragile; I felt as if I was drowning and needed desperately to find a lifeline because I wanted to die and could no longer hang on. The only energy I could muster up was enough to barely take care of my girls, (my son had moved in with my husband). I knew that I had to be strong for my girls even though I was so weak and my heart was in so much pain. Each school day I would take my girls to school in my pajamas only to immediately return home to lie on my couch to cry, be sad and unproductive until it was time to pick them up, still in my pajamas. This unhealthiness went on for many weeks.

The first of many pivotal moments for me was when I laid on the shower floor in the fetal position crying in utter pain and sheer confusion trying to figure out how my life had been turned upside down and flipped inside out, especially since I was a "good Christian." I couldn't understand how the God I "gave" my life to, could allow this to happen to me and how dare He let me go through so much suffering. As I laid on the ground demanding God to answer my questions and brazenly reminding Him of who I was and all that I did for Him, I came to the realization, a revelation; that I had lost everything and I was now at a place of complete nothingness. I had been broken down to extinction: I had no identity, I had no material things, I could no longer do it by myself, I was weak, I was tired, I was beaten down, I had no more fight in me, I was nobody and I had nobody, I was abandoned, I had no hope and worse, I could see no hope. I had succumbed to my very last option; surrender and yield to what God was offering. Surrender meant that I had to abdicate everything if I wanted to live again. I had only enough strength left to barely mumble the words, "Help me please God" as I laid there in my prostrate position begging repeatedly until it was only a faint phrase that was mimicked only by my lips and no more sound. In that very moment of pleading, complete peace came over me, a peace that surpassed all of my understanding. Silence filled the bathroom and the loud clamoring of the chaos of my circumstances ceased to exist, and the only thing I could hear was my breath ricocheting off of the shower floor as I felt my chest rise and fall with each sob. God was there with me, in the midst of all my turmoil, He hadn't left me.

As the days passed, the meek little fighter inside of me finally rose up and said, "This is enough and my children deserved more than this from me." Something needed to change because I was spiraling downward quickly and with every passing day, I would lose more hope. So I set my mind, I made a decision, a choice, to get off of the couch and to carry myself to the gym, if for anything, to just change my scenery.

At the gym, I walked on the treadmill crying, still desperately trying to understand how I lost everything, and why what I did and who I was wasn't enough. The revelation of having no identity, no self-esteem, no self worth, no value left me completely lost, confused, and scared. The pain from the feeling of abandonment has helped me to understand why many would contemplate suicide, because I did.

I believe the very worse thing any one person can ever experience in life is the feeling of abandonment, no matter what form it comes in. To feel like you're unworthy, invaluable, unlovable, and not worth fighting for, leaves deep wounds that many are unable to be revived from.

My choice to not take my own life laid in the awareness that I wasn't the only one who was hurting. My babies were going through the same pain and their pain was probably at a deeper level because they did not understand or were capable of comprehending why their world had changed so drastically. The insight of this left me with no other choice but to fight for them, to assure them that I would never abandon them and to show them that they were indeed worth fighting for and **I**, their mother, would be that fighter who would fight for them <u>even</u> <u>if</u> nobody was fighting for me. The unwavering love I had for my children brought me to a place where I had NO option but to be strong for them. I knew the importance in how I chose to deal with and react to this provisional time of torment was going to leave an impacting impression upon them and would absolutely influence the outcome of their lives.

To learn that the life of another is dependent on you is not only a serious responsibility but also a terrifying one.

When you are forsaken by someone you love, your internal desire to understand why you weren't good enough often times leads you to wanting somebody, maybe anybody, to fill the void that you feel. I had this desire and though I had my girls, I was still lonely. I often missed the feeling of security that came with my husband's hugs. I also missed being kissed and even just the touch of his hand. I just wanted to feel a man's hand on my skin because it had been so long since I had been touched, not in a sexual way but to just feel the touch of another on my skin. I deplorably made an appointment for a one-hour massage at the spa with a male massage therapist. As I lay there mournful upon the massage table in the dimly lit room, tears streamed down my face, I thought to myself, "How pathetic are you to have to pay for a massage just so you can feel the touch of another human?" I was thankful for the lack of light in the dimly lit room because it hid my tears and the chilled room temperature was the explanation I gave to the massage therapist for my sniffling, when he asked if I was all right.

Though my heart was severely broken and I was very lonely I quickly noticed that though my husband no longer wanted me, there were many men wanting and vying to fill his vacancy, all claiming to be knights in shining armor; I did not want any of it or any of them. I didn't want to be like my husband or all of the other people I watched go through break ups only to enter another unsuccessful one for selfish needs. I didn't want or need another person to fill my void. Not to mention, how selfish it would be of me to run to another man to fulfill my needs with nothing to offer back to him. I knew that any relationship that I would enter into would be doomed before it began because I would've brought unprofitable baggage into the relationship. I would have taken more than I was giving to the relationship because I had nothing left to give; everything had been stolen from me. I knew that **I needed to fix me**, I needed to heal, I wanted to heal and I needed to learn who I was and in the end I wanted a relationship with someone who complimented me, not one that was suppose to complete me. So I chose to chase God and not men.

God took me unconditionally just where I was, promising to give me everything I needed though I came with empty hands. He accepted me just as I was: emotionally broken, spiritually vulnerable, physically flaccid and mentally exhausted.

At this time, I was in the burrows so I chose to dig tunnels within God's word every weekend that my girls spent away with their dad. I thought I knew who God was but I was determined to try to learn more about who He really was and what He was about. During my search, I discovered who I was and more importantly who I was to God. I learned that the God who had created this earth and all things did so with a purpose and with so much beauty distinctively for my pleasure, my enjoyment and my benefit, not missing any detail. He intently created beauty for me to experience in every aspect of my life because He loved me so very much and desired to give me His very best because I was special to Him. I also learned that he created beauty within me. He had a plan and a purpose for my life and had already pre-equipped me with the tools I needed to achieve it, I only needed to trust Him, and believe that with Him what seemed impossible was actually possible.

In one of the many quiet times I spent with God, I distinctly remember Him saying to me, "Alysia, why are you being so pitiful? I did not make you to be pitiful. I made you to be great, to go do great things for your life and to let the beauty that was inside of you out for others to see, all for My name's sake. Stop being what you are not and boldly be what I created you to be. Go audaciously and enjoy and experience what I created for you. The gifts and talents that you have, I planted in you when you were young, remember those things that made your heart smile and do that. It is those things that will help you step into the purpose for which I intentionally created you for." Then God asked me, "Do you think I would have allowed this to happen to you if it were going to keep you from your destiny, from My will for your life? Your identity is <u>NOT</u> in your husband, but in Me. I gave you this life to live amazingly for My glory. I planted the seeds (your talents and skills) to your success deep within you. The dreams I gave you, as a child is what you're suppose to do with your life. So REMEMBER!"

As I listened, I tried to remember what brought me joy in my youth, what made my heart sing. I went over my lost bucket list and reminded myself of all of the things I wanted to see, visit, and experience in my life before I died.

This moment of my journey God challenged and provoked me with three questions:

1.) Am I who I want to be?
2.) Is my life everything I dreamed that it would be?
3.) Will I be courageous enough to find out?"

As a young girl having come from a dysfunctional and abusive home, left me with the longing for what I thought love was. Watching my parents and others, I knew that I did not want to love as they did, instead I wanted to love unconditionally and I wanted to be loved unconditionally. So I set out determined to accomplish this desire of my heart.

Once God told me to stop being pitiful; I set my mind and I started paying attention to the beauty around me. I dusted off my bucket list and I went over it, adding a few more things to it. I remembered the big crazy unfathomable dreams I had as a young girl and then I decided to start scratching things off of my list. I began to invest into me and into my children. I made time to read more and watch less television, I spent more time with my babies, I made a point to cherish and appreciate the people who loved me, I prayed a lot, I spent much of my time with God, talking to Him throughout my day. I gave away to others what I needed most. God showed me that, if I wanted love, I must first give love, if I want understanding I must seek to understand, if I wanted kindness I needed to be kind. I intentionally set my number one goal to be healing and to achieve one of my childhood dreams, the dream of real unconditional love.

The break down of my relationship with my husband left my emotional bank account bankrupt once again and I needed love just as much as I needed a vacation. I can remember talking to God about this. I informed Him, though He already knew, that I needed something, I wanted to feel love and I needed a break from my broken heart. I had no money to get away although I needed to badly. I knew that if I did get to go on vacation I would come back with only more debt, a tan and nothing else to show for it. God answered this prayer in a unique way and took care of both needs for me; sending me on my first mission trip to Nicaragua, a trip that was not only very fulfilling but began the healing of my heart. Upon my return from my trip, I joined a women's Bible study aboard the Marine Corps Base, they were studying the book of Esther. This study had a powerful impact on the way I lived my life and set my mind on a course that helped lead me to where I am now. Throughout the study I learned that I had much in common, with Esther and I easily related greatly to her. Esther's fearlessness in the face of fear nurtured the audacious fighter that existed within me and invited this fighter to boldly come out in a fierce and fearless way.

The people we love are only in our lives for a short time, some shorter than others.

I not only had the desire to discover who I was but an obligation to. In doing so, I not only unveiled that there were many lessons that I still needed to learn in order to know myself better, to mature more but also to grow in character. One lesson I learned and took away from my divorce was an all-powerful one; what it meant to truly appreciate and love those who unquestionably mattered to me in a tenacious way. I learned how to love and appreciate others in their love language and not with mine (Read the 5 Love Languages by Dr. Gary Chapman). With each new friendship God placed on my path I diligently sought to learn the true meaning of what love meant; valuing people, making the most of the time I got to spend with them, not taking them or our time together for granted and to leave them feeling valued. God taught me the importance of always being in the moment with those I chose to spend my time with, to fearlessly be vulnerable when I tell the people who mattered most to me how I felt about them and what they meant to me, despite the chance of being rejected again. I mindfully practiced being patient, accountable, not keeping records or hold grudges, and to look for the best in others while always attempting to first seek to understand before trying to be understood. I became overzealous, loving with reckless abandon. Living this way I know I will never regret, though many think I am weird because of it.

As I went through my bucket list, I chose bodybuilding as the first dream I wanted to accomplish. Each day after I dropped my girls off to school, I would head to the gym. While at the gym, I would talk to God during my cardio session and then I would work out on the machines listening to sermons and the same songs I have written in the workout at the end of this book. I graduated from walking on the treadmill to being able to run on it. During my workouts I listened closely to the words God spoke to me through the songs and sermons.

Finally, I decided to compete in a body building competition, I needed to share my decision. Once I got past the fear of announcing my idea to my friends, I shared publicly, posting it on Facebook making it official (ha-ha, because we all know that it just isn't "official" until it's posted on Facebook). I needed an accountability partner and my Facebook friends became that.

Once I announced my decision to compete, God then started strategically placing people in my life and on my path to help me, to teach me, to guide me. Like always, He didn't just send just anyone to help me, He sent me the best. He didn't just give me a trainer He gave me a PNBA (Professional Natural Bodybuilding Association) pro bodybuilder to help me get to my goal of competing.

I trained long and hard, always focusing, practicing discipline and training not only my body but also my mind. I followed a strict diet and training plan. I got up early, I trained often and I grew stronger in all aspects of my life; I lost the excess weight and baggage both from my body and in my life: physically I got stronger, more defined and shed the pounds, mentally I became more determined and goal oriented, spiritually I grew closer to God, and emotionally I became invincible, nothing anybody said to me could effect me any longer, I knew who I was and whose I was. I became unstoppable.

On my 40th birthday, I stepped onto a stage in front of an audience filled with hundreds of people to include my two daughters. I knew that when I walked out into the spotlight I would not only be revealing the muscles I gained and my new fit figure but more importantly, I would be showcasing all of my hard work, my perseverance, a year of all that I had endured, all that I had to overcome to get there and most importantly, I would be sharing three messages; the first was to my daughters. The first message would teach and prove to them that we do not have to be a victim of our circumstances but instead we can choose to be the victor and with much hard work, determination, and faith in God we would overcome. The next message was confirmation of my promise to them that I would ALWAYS fearlessly fight for them, that I would preserve no matter what came at me. My third message was a reminder to myself and now to you; the exhibition of two of the many promises God made to me and He makes to you; "All things do work together for the good to those who love God, to those who are called according to HIS purpose." (Romans 8:28 ESV) and "Blessed is she who has believed that the Lord would fulfill His promises to her." (Luke 1:45 NIV) On that stage, I not only showcased my transformation in every aspect of my life but I shared my heart as I stood proud and tall upon that stage.

Whether I won or not didn't really honestly matter to me. I knew that even if I didn't place or get to hold a trophy in my hand that day, I knew that God was holding me up as His trophy. Me being on that stage was ALL for His glory and not for mine. I knew God, my potter, was holding me up in His right hand saying, "Look at her, Alysia, my beautiful and precious girl, look what I did for her and to her. Look at her transformation into the beautiful masterpiece that she always was." Being on that stage God showed me that I could overcome as long as I stayed in faith, kept my eyes on the prize, and if I kept fighting with no excuses. I walked off that stage a winner, having come out stronger and undefeatable in all areas of my life.

I didn't know just how strong I really was until I was at my breaking point; broken, weak, crying out to God and holding onto Him as if my life depended on it, in the end, it did. My choice to listen to God and to answer those provoked challenge questions He pose to me led me to the path of bodybuilding, I learned so much and like everything, it came at the perfect time, at the appointed time, in His time. God used bodybuilding as the vehicle to teach me more about discipline, about focus and determination and pushing past the pain, not just physically but mentally, emotionally, and spiritually. I slowly regained my self-esteem and my self-confidence. My training not only made me physically stronger but it mentally taught me that my mind controls my body and NOT the pain (this did not just mean the physical pain but the mental and emotional pain that I was enduring). I grew closer to God each day as well with each prayer. As each day passed, God made me more capable and able, He would place random people to include strangers on my path to tell me I was beautiful, to tell me I was strong, and to tell me I was special. God taught me how to love myself for the first time in my life and He brought me to a place where I liked me.

Like a piece of clay pottery, God picked up my broken pieces and put them through the very hot furnace and remolded me. He transformed not only my mind and my body but also my heart and He lifted the veil from my eyes. He told me who I was and whose I was. He showed me that He would fight for me and that I was worthy, valuable, and precious to Him. He kept every promise He made to me and He never left me—He never abandoned me and He loved me, HE was the one who fought for me, He was the one who chose me when no other wanted me.

"We love him because he first loved us."
1 John 4:19 (KJV)

It was God who first loved me. I've been called a Jesus fanatic and I don't mind it because from that very moment of me crying out to God, He proved to me that He had never left me and never would when everyone else did even when I was unfaithful to Him. God was the only one who kept every promise ever made to me; always making a way for my children and me even when there seemed to be no way—he fed me, he housed me, he helped me. Throughout this journey God rebuilt me, showed me my value, He gave me back my worth and a new identity, He placed the most amazing people in my life and placed people on my path that would help me as well as challenge me. He gave me back my dreams, desires and then some; giving me hope and showing me I had a life worth living. He gave me a new reason to live and to exist. He took the anger, bitterness, and hate that was filling my heart and he replaced it with a genuine LOVE that I cannot keep contained nor keep from others. He transformed my mind, my heart, and my eyes, giving me compassionate eyes and understanding to see those who are unkind to me the way He sees them. He worked forgiveness into my heart that set me free. He not only told me I was beautiful but showed me the beauty that I could not see. He told me I was worth something to Him, that I was the "crown of His creation."(Captivating, Staci and John Eldridge) He took my shattered and broken pieces and He sculpted them back together through testing and trials and created a new confident, strong, loving and more beautiful woman who now knows that she is worthy to be healed, loved and fought for. Just like a potter does when he molds pieces of clay together before putting it through the fire.

God set me on fire and then He let me loose, His new creation that had always been hidden inside but needed refining before being placed back into the world; a zealous bold woman with a burning desire to recklessly love the people on her path and in her life while living the most incredible life, proving to her girls that they are worth fighting for while desiring and aspiring to give hope and inspiration to others while chasing the dreams He planted within. How does the saying go? "It's the people who are crazy enough to think they can change the world--are the ones who do." My hope is that I am one of those crazy people. I try to live my life in a way that each person that I encounter will know that they are valuable just because they exist. I may not be able to do much for them, but I can share the truth about hope, I can make them feel the love of God that pours from my heart for them and if it's only but a brief moment of our encounter, my goal is always to leave God-prints in their lives when I leave.

After my bodybuilding competition, I went on to get a teaching credential with the state of California so that I could become a substitute teacher, enabling me to teach children of all ages. During my classroom times, I try to teach the students at least one life lesson, whether it be about respect, accountability, kindness, understanding, character, forgiveness or to just tell them that they can chase their dreams if they are willing to fight and believe in themselves. The very thing God taught me.

A few months after receiving my teaching credential, I revisited my bucket list, and finished getting my personal trainer certification. I not only teach in a classroom setting to young students, I now train clients in the gym. I not only transform their bodies, but I teach them how to train their minds, pushing them past their pain, to step out and try something they didn't think they could ever do, and I edify them by reminding them if not tell them that they are stronger than they know.

My path has been filled and continues to be filled with many blessings from God and will continue to be; I was given the opportunity to step on the stage to perform a comedy set that I wrote in front of a large audience, I picked up two body building sponsors, I have been invited to many red carpet events, God has allowed my path to cross with many professional athletes, celebrities and also people from around the world whom I do not know but who reach out to me asking me to pray for them, encourage them or to give them just a little bit of hope.

Though my journey through the desert was torturous and lonely, I am thankful that I got to be the vessel that God chose to use for the benefit of not just me, but hopefully for many others. I am thankful that God has given me a platform to share my testimony to many and my prayer is that it gives hope and inspiration for anyone who needs it or even a glimpse of light at the end of a dark tunnel for someone who desperately needs one but most importantly, I hope people will come to know the God who rescued me through my actions, my words, and my life and I am praying that He will also become a cistern of living water to those who are hurting and thirsty for love and healing.

A humble gratefulness overflows from my heart because from each instance and trial I learned something, I became a better person, I was given the opportunity to grow, to gain more character, to become more accepting, to love others unconditionally and the chances to prove to God that I can be trusted with what He has given to me. It is because of the pain, suffering and heartache that I endured that I am stronger and more focused. I am determined, I am fearless, I am confident, I am bold and I am alive. I was blind, but now I see, I was lost but now I'm found. I've been made new. I've been set on a new path clothed in strength and dignity, laughing without fear at the future. I know whose I am and I desire all that He has for me, all that He has promised me; and I WILL receive it ALL.

I'm excited about deepening the relationships I have now and I look forward to the new relationships that I will start with the people who are daring enough to get to know me. I'm jumping in with all that I have, and I'm not looking back. With my faith, I will leap. As I once wrote, I am purposefully coloring outside of the lines of my dreams with my life so sit back and watch…I'm going to be conquering goal after goal, chasing dream after dream, kicking butt and taking names and you can rest assure, I will be doing it in lip gloss, high heels with a six pack of abs!

So again, with a thankful and humble heart, I must give praise and glory first and foremost to my ever so REAL and present faithful God, my provider, my protector and my sculptor. Thank you for never leaving me or forsaking me. Thanking you for your provisions and faithfulness and Redemptive LOVE.

* * * * * * * * * * * * * * * * * * * *

My husband (now ex-husband) is not my enemy nor a bad person at heart, he's deceived, battling his own demons, and he like all of us, got lost somewhere along the way and is now trying to find his way, so my heart has absolutely NO resentment, unforgiveness, or hate for or towards him. Being the father of our three amazing children, he will always hold his own place in my heart.

Lastly, thank you to all of those who betrayed me, abandoned me, used me, took advantage of me and hurt me whether it was a spoken word or comment or just out of pure meanness, those who gossiped and lied about me and made me the butt of their jokes, who mocked me, slandered my name and character to people who did and others that didn't know me, to those who didn't keep their word to me and to those who hoped that it would be the end of me... all of it made me stronger and better, it caused me to constantly challenge myself, to try harder, it tested my will and my character, it motivated me and most of all, it has empowered me. Please know that I have forgiven you.

* * * * * * * * * * * * * * * * * * * *

So as I say goodbye to the end of this portion of my life, I'm going to continue moving forward with eyes, arms and heart wide open, determined and focused but more importantly fearlessly. This season is not only literally a chapter in this book I have been writing for you but now a mere chapter in my past. I'm not closing the book I'm simply turning the page and ready to write the next chapter as well as the next book. As much as I wanted to plan my life, it had an amazing way of surprising me with the unexpected things and turn of events that not only made me happier and encouraged me to become better than I ever planned, imagined or hoped for—this was God's will for my life and I consciously choose to step into it every morning when I open my eyes with a joyful, thankful and expectant heart. My desire and prayer is that

I have been able to give hope and inspire those of you that may have needed it, not just with my words but with the way I have chosen to live my life.

For those of you who have been and who are still struggling, with addictions, betrayal, unforgiveness, and hopelessness I can testify that this too shall come to pass. Cry out to the One that can change your circumstances and take what He has to offer for free, it's so much better than anything you could ever imagine. Remember that we are here but for a brief moment, our life goes quickly and we only get one chance to make the most of every day, of every opportunity and of every relationship because time is the one thing we cannot get back, once it's gone, it's gone. Learn and grow from your trials, remove the unhealthy and or abusive people or relationships from your life, always speak positively especially in your darkest moments, consciously be in the moment of every moment and bravely choose to feel every emotion and don't forget your dreams, but rather, CHASE THEM RELENTLESSLY!

Know that if God did it for me; He <u>wants</u>, He <u>can</u> and He <u>will</u> do it for you! **God Loves You more than you can Fathom!**

It's time, it's <u>your</u> time, it's **FOR SUCH A TIME AS THIS!**

Thank you for taking the time and effort to walk with me through my journey, listening to my heart and most intimate thoughts and for reading my testimony - this book, my book, that I wrote for you; FOR SUCH A TIME AS THIS. May God bless you and may you fulfill the amazing purpose for which you were created. Your talents, skills, and blessings were given to you to share with the world...go do it, and do it fearlessly, you victorious overcomer!

Chapter 9

REPENTANCE

*"Repent, then, and turn to God, so that your sins may be
wiped out, that times of refreshing may come from the Lord"
Acts 3:19 (NIV)*

No one is happier than when they have sincerely repented for their wrongs. Repentance is the decision to turn from our selfish desires and turn the other way, never looking back. It is a genuine, sincere regret that creates sorrow that moves us to admit our wrongs giving us the desire to do better and to be better, to become new.

Genuine repentance is a moving condition of the heart that is testified and demonstrated by our deeds. It's an inward conviction that expresses itself with outward actions.

You look at the love of God and you can't believe He's loved you like He has, and it motivates you to change your life. That is the nature of repentance.

My pivotal moment through my entire life, the moment I learned what true repentance was, what it truly meant, and what it felt like took place on that shower floor in my bathroom. That was the moment that God didn't just wipe away my discrepancies but cloaked me in his robe of righteousness and the transformation of my heart began. It was the moment I began to turn away from old ways, I placed all of my burdens at the foot of the cross and received everything God was offering.

Truth: God loves you so very much that He gave his only son to give His life for you (John 3:16). Jesus came to this earth and lived as a sinless man and was betrayed, lied to, mistreated, abused and then as an innocent man was crucified by his haters and was hung on a cross and shed His blood. He died and rose from the dead three days later. Jesus Christ IS the son of God and it is only when you believe this and you confess it with your mouth and ask for His forgiveness can you have all of your wrong doings, your iniquities, your shortcomings, your dark secrets etc. be forgiven and wiped away to be replaced with God's love, His blessings, and everything He has for you. Instead of mocking this or questioning it, why not believe that you are worthy of being loved, that the God who breathed life into all things finds you special and important to Him. Who wants you and wants to have a relationship with you, who chooses YOU. Why be cynical when it's easier to say, thank you and take His love and adoration and accept it. For once, remove your thoughts and trust this truth I share with you, ignore your doubts and just take what God wants to give to you so freely because you matter to Him. You say you need proof, my life that I am sharing with you intimately is proof, these words I have written in this book for you are true.

I didn't choose or want the suffering of my life or the way the path of my journey started but I am genuinely thankful to where it has led and where it is going. I can honestly say that the darkest moments of this recent part of my journey upon this earth became the catalyst that made me choose to cry out to my Creator. It was this one choice that catapulted me into the amazing life I now get to live. If you would like to ask God into your life, into your situation, to help you change, to help you heal, to help you go from broken to blessed, to help you step into your destiny taking everything He has for you, with a sincere desiring heart I would like to encourage you to faithfully pray this prayer out loud.

Dear God,

I am hurting right now. I believe that you do love me and you do want and have good things for me. I do believe that you sent your only son, Jesus Christ, to die and shed his blood for me then rising from the grave three days later. I confess that Jesus Christ is your son and I want you to come into my life, into my situation and to help me. Forgive me of my wrong doings, and help me to forgive those who have hurt me, and to help me to forgive myself. I want you to heal every part of me and set me free. I want a life filled with joy, peace, and hope. I want everything that you did for Alysia; I want you to do it for me. I want to walk in your favor, to receive your grace and mercy, and I want your blessings. Change my heart, my mind, and my body. Make me into what you created me to be, a victorious overcomers. I thank you now for hearing and answering my prayer and from this day forward, I pledge to You to serve you all the days of my life. May Your will be done in my life. I pray this believing all of these things will come to pass. In your son's precious, powerful and transforming name. Amen.

If you prayed this prayer with a sincere heart, you have now been saved and your name is now written in God's book of life, you are now a member of God's family and warrior in His army. Your flaws, shortcomings, failures, and sins have been wiped away and you are now cloaked in God's robe of righteousness. God will begin to move in you life, in your situation, and in your heart. Find a church, get a Bible and read it daily, watch a video or listen to an audio Christian sermon often. Continue to chase God relentlessly even when things get hard, just because you became a Christian does not mean life will get easier but it will get better and watch what amazing things He does for you and with your life. He did it for me and **I promise**, **if you chase Him, especially in your darkest times, God will keep all of His promises to you** and do for you what He did for me. You matter to Him, He loves you and He wants to give you all that He has for you. Remember, being a Christian is about having a close personal relationship with Jesus Christ, it's not about religion or having a must do list or traditions, it's about spending time with God praying, talking to Him daily, inviting Him into all aspects of your life and spending time reading His word (the Bible).

> *Almighty God, Creator of All Things,*
>
> *I come boldly before your throne of mercy and grace and I give you praise and honor and I thank you for your son Jesus Christ. I lift up every person who has read my story and I stand in the gap for them asking you to move in their lives and in their situation in a mighty and powerful way. Transform them and their hearts and bring them to a place of healing and peace and freedom, all of the things your precious Son died for to give to them. I ask that your Holy Spirit move within their hearts and that their hearts and mind are open and receptive to you and your calling on their lives. I ask for your blessings upon them. Plant in them a desire to seek you more and the courage to step out in faith boldly. Bring them people to speak life into their lives giving them hope and a desire for more. I pray that my words have spoken to their hearts and that they choose to take all that you have for them, to be free, to fight for peace, to be victorious overcomers. May Your will be done in each of their lives. I thank you for having already gone before them and for answering this prayer. In Jesus' healing name I pray. Amen. Amen. Amen.*

My Princess...
ASK ME ANYTHING

I am all-powerful, and I am preparing you for something significant in My eternal plan. Don't be afraid to dream big just because of past disappointments. Remember, it wasn't your faith in *Me* that failed you, it was your faith in people that caused the pain of broken dreams. I am your King, and I can do anything you ask in My name. King David started out as a small shepherd boy, but had faith big enough to kill a giant. I am just as real today in *you* as I was back then. So ask Me, obey Me, and seek Me with all your heart, mind, and strength. And then watch My promises to you come to pass in my perfect time.

Love,

Your King and Answer to everything

This is a picture of a message God gave to me as a promise before my life began to fall apart. He spoke to me long before I knew anything was going to happen. Today, as I finish this book, I came across this picture; it was God's reminder to me on this day that He did indeed keep His promises to me. My heart smiles at the ways in which God speaks to me as well as the divine nature of His timing.

This picture, is of the card that I wrote to myself after the Esther study. Our group leader gave us each a blank card and told us to write ourselves a message, which she would mail a few weeks later. She ended up moving, misplacing the cards and mailing them later than planned. On the exact day the girls and I moved into our new apartment to begin our new life, the card arrived in the mail. As I sat alone having no recollection of what I had written on the last day of the study, I opened the card and began to read. Tears began to run down my cheek as I realized that every word I had written was true and had come to pass. I was amazed and in awe with God's impeccable timing, it came exactly when I needed to read it.

Chapter 10

EXPLANATION OF WORKOUT

The workout I have written is not just a physical workout. It is mental training as well. My program is designed to not only transform your body but your mind as well as the way you think, the way you see yourself, leaving you with a new outlook on life. You will be more confident, empowered, and strong minded at the end of the 30-day workout. The steps I share in the workout are the exact steps God took me through to take me from broken to blessed. You will be transformed from the inside out after 30 days of my program and you will be on a new course for your life, a course that will lead you straight into the destiny you were created to live.

MUSIC: The songs I have included in the workout are for you to meditate on. Listen to the words of each song as you workout. Listen to them as you pray. Listen to them as you go through your day. Music is an important instrument that helps in the healing process as well as the transformation process. For 30 days, ONLY listen to the songs on my song list or on Christian radio, do your best not to listen to other music. This is an important part of the 30-day plan for your success.

PRAYER: Prayer is vital in so many ways. It not only allows you to speak to God it helps you to vent, it opens your heart to the hearing of what God has to say to you. The more you pray the more you will hear what God has to say with you. This will help you feel more secure, builds your faith, increase your realization of who you are and whose you are. The beginning of the month's workout you will pray novice prayers. I wrote these as a guideline for those who don't know how to pray or what to pray. As you continue on through the program your prayers will grow from uncertain to faithful. The prayers will help you get ready for the next level of your journey. In the end you will have a closer personal relationship with God and if you are an unbeliever, you will learn that the God I serve is real and He loves and cares for you as much as He loves me. If you are an unbeliever, I am asking you to give it a try for only 30 days and then decide on day 31.

SPEAK LIFE: The words we speak have a lot to do with the way we see ourselves, the way we feel about ourselves, and it determines our level of self-esteem. The words that have been spoken over us have played a part of the way we feel, the way we think about ourselves, and the way we see ourselves. The words we speak play an important factor in the outcome of our future. There is power in the words we speak and in the words spoken to us. I have given you words to speak to help condition your mind, to teach you and to tell you who you are. I want you to know whose you are and how valuable you are to God and to empower you. When words are played over and over in our minds and we hear it over and over, the words soon drop from our mind to our heart, once in our heart it becomes who we are. Write the Speak Life words on a sticky note each day and stick the sticky note somewhere you can see it. Whenever you see one of the sticky notes, you must read it out loud. I have done this to deprogram the negative words that play in your mind about yourself and to reprogram the way you see yourself, the way you were created to be.

STRETCHING: Stretching is an essential part of fitness and in health. I've included stretches that will help with each day's workout. I've included directions on how to do the stretches at the end of this book. Or visit my YouTube channel: Alysia Rieg

THE WORKOUT: The workout is designed to train your body to do what it needs to do to transform; not just for size but for your health. You will lose fat and gain muscle while you gain more self-confidence and a greater self-esteem level. At the end of the program you will see that your body has transformed from the inside out. When the 30 days is over, I would like to encourage you to continue following the program and working out. Please email me at forsuchatimeasthisbook@gmail.com or at teamalysia@gmail.com and tell me about your 30 day journey.

Things you Need:
- Bible
- Highlighter & Pen
- Sticky Notes
- Notebook
- Workout Program
- Measuring Tape
- Ipod / MP3 Player
- Water
- Towel

Things to Do:
- Take before picture (front, sides, back) Every month take new pictures.
- **EMAIL ME YOUR BEFORE AND AFTER PICTURES: forsuchatimeasthisbook@gmail.com or at teamalysia@gmail.com**

In the subject line write, For Such A Time As This Workout Before and After Pictures

- Measure (use the measurement chart provided) Take measurements every month.
- Put music on Ipod or MP3 player (see song list)
- Try your BEST to follow workout program EXACTLY
- WORKOUT, SWEAT, HAVE FUN, GET STRONGER IN MANY WAYS and GROW

To see my transformation picture, my before and after pictures, visit my website: alysiarieg.com or my Instagram: ay_lee_see_yuh or my Facebook Page: Alysia Rieg (athlete)

MEASURE: (on Day 1 and Day 31)

Date:

Neck: _____   Chest: _____   Waist: _____   Hips: _____

L Thigh: _____   R Thigh: _____   L Bicep: _____   R Bicep: _____

L Calf: _____   R Calf: _____   L Wrist: _____   R Wrist: _____

Date:

Neck: _____   Chest: _____   Waist: _____   Hips: _____

L Thigh: _____   R Thigh: _____   L Bicep: _____   R Bicep: _____

L Calf: _____   R Calf: _____   L Wrist: _____   R Wrist: _____

Chapter 11

FOR SUCH A TIME AS THIS
30 DAY WORKOUT

* Consult a doctor before doing this or any workout program. *

THINGS TO REMEMBER

- Make a new SPEAK LIFE sticky note for each session and hang it where you can see it and say it aloud.
- Play the songs listed for each workout on repeat during each session.
- If the day has 2 sessions, you will workout 2 times that day. Preferably in the a.m. and then in the p.m.
- Do the workout in order.
- Pray during cardio sessions and during stretching sessions. Prayers are listed in workout. *(Write notes in your notebook during this time as you feel.)*
- Increase speed and incline as instructed.
- Continue the previous speed and incline until instructed to increase.
- Stretch before and after each workout. Stretches are listed in workout. (See the Stretch Section of the Book for stretch instructions.)

- Hold each stretch for at least: Warm Up 10-20 seconds, Post Workout 30-45 seconds.
- Don't forget your water, a towel, your notebook, a pen, your headphones and music from song list. (Songs for each workout is listed in workout.)

✓ *Note: Listen closely to the words of each song.*
✓ *Note: It is alright to cry during the workout. Crying is an essential part of healing.*
✓ *Note: If you don't know how to do some of the exercises, search them on my YouTube Channel: Alysia Rieg or my website:* **alysiarieg.com**

Dear God,

Please use this workout to make my body physically capable for whatever tasks You need me to accomplish. Make it more than just fat-burning, calorie blasting, or cellulite shedding. Let this workout be an action that shows my heart's openness and willingness to serve You whenever and wherever You need me. Let the results of my transformation prove to everyone that it was You who transformed me from the inside out. In Jesus' name I pray. Amen. Amen. Amen.

DAY 1 SESSION 1

WARM UP STRETCHES Hold 10 - 20 seconds each	SPEAK LIFE I am going to be alright.	SONG LISTS FOR:
CARDIO	**PRAYER**	**STRETCHING** Oceans, Hillsong United
Treadmill: 30– 60 minutes Incline: 0 Beginning Speed: 0 – 2.0 **POST WORKOUT STRETCHES** Hold 30 - 45 seconds each: Calf Stretch Hamstring Stretch IT Band Stretch Kneeling Runners Pose Quadriceps Stretch Sciatic Stretch	-Ask God why. -Tell God what you think. -Tell God what you feel. -Tell God what you want. -Thank God for what you have.	**CARDIO** Before the Morning, Josh Wilson Broken, Lifehouse Call My Name, Third Day Can Anybody Hear Me, Meredith Andrews Cry Out To Jesus, Third Day Held, Natalie Grant Hold My Heart, Tenth Avenue North I Need A Miracle, Third Day

DAY 1 SESSION 2

WARM UP STRETCHES Hold 10 - 20 seconds each	SPEAK LIFE I am special.	SONG LISTS FOR:
CARDIO	**PRAYER**	STRETCHING Oceans, Hillsong United
Treadmill: 30–60 minutes Incline: 0 Speed: _____ **POST WORKOUT STRETCHES** Hold 30 - 45 seconds each: Calf Stretch Hamstring Stretch IT Band Stretch Kneeling Runners Pose Quadriceps Stretch Sciatic Stretch	-Ask God why. -Tell God what you think. -Tell God what you feel. -Tell God what you want. -Thank God for what you have.	**CARDIO** Before the Morning, Josh Wilson Broken, Lifehouse Call My Name, Third Day Can Anybody Hear Me, Meredith Andrews Cry Out To Jesus, Third Day Held, Natalie Grant Hold My Heart, Tenth Avenue North I Need A Miracle, Third Day

DAY 2 SESSION 1

WARM UP STRETCHES Hold 10 - 20 seconds each	SPEAK LIFE I am important.	SONG LISTS FOR:	
CARDIO	PRAYER	Oceans, Hillsong United	STRETCHING
Treadmill: 30–60 minutes Incline: 1 - 1.5 Speed: _____	-Ask God why. -Tell God what you think. -Tell God what you feel. -Tell God what you want. -Thank God for what you have.	Before the Morning, Josh Wilson Broken, Lifehouse Call My Name, Third Day Can Anybody Hear Me, Meredith Andrews Cry Out To Jesus, Third Day Held, Natalie Grant Hold My Heart, Tenth Avenue North I Need A Miracle, Third Day	CARDIO
POST WORKOUT STRETCHES Hold 30 - 45 seconds each: Calf Stretch Hamstring Stretch IT Band Stretch Kneeling Runners Pose Quadriceps Stretch Sciatic Stretch			

DAY 2 SESSION 2

WARM UP STRETCHES Hold 10 - 20 seconds each	SPEAK LIFE I am beautiful.	SONG LISTS FOR:	
CARDIO	PRAYER	Oceans, Hillsong United	STRETCHING
Treadmill: 30–60 minutes Incline: 1 – 1.5 Speed: _____	-Ask God why. -Tell God what you think. -Tell God what you feel. -Tell God what you want. -Thank God for what you have.	I Loved You Then, 33 Miles Jesus Loves Me, Chris Tomlin Jesus Heals Your Heart, Third Day Love Is Not A Fight, Warren Barfield Love Never Fails, Brandon Heath Remind Me Who I Am, Jason Gray Unfailing Love, Chris Tomlin	CARDIO
POST WORKOUT STRETCHES Hold 30 - 45 seconds each: Calf Stretch Hamstring Stretch IT Band Stretch Kneeling Runners Pose Quadriceps Stretch Sciatic Stretch			

DAY 3 SESSION 1

WARM UP STRETCHES Hold 10 - 20 seconds each	SPEAK LIFE I matter.	SONG LISTS FOR:
		STRETCHING
CARDIO	PRAYER	Oceans, Hillsong United
Treadmill: 30–60 minutes Incline: 2 – 2.5 Speed:_____ POST WORKOUT STRETCHES Hold 30 - 45 seconds each: Calf Stretch Hamstring Stretch IT Band Stretch Kneeling Runners Pose Quadriceps Stretch Sciatic Stretch	-Ask God why. -Tell God what you think. -Tell God what you feel. -Tell God what you want. -Thank God for what you have.	CARDIO I Loved You Then, 33 Miles Jesus Loves Me, Chris Tomlin Jesus Heals Your Heart, Third Day Love Is Not A Fight, Warren Barfield Love Never Fails, Brandon Heath Remind Me Who I Am, Jason Gray Unfailing Love, Chris Tomlin

DAY 2 SESSION 2

WARM UP STRETCHES Hold 10 - 20 seconds each	SPEAK LIFE I am beautiful.	SONG LISTS FOR:
		STRETCHING
CARDIO	PRAYER	Oceans, Hillsong United
Treadmill: 30–60 minutes Incline: 2 – 2.5 Speed:_____ POST WORKOUT STRETCHES Hold 30 - 45 seconds each: Calf Stretch Hamstring Stretch IT Band Stretch Kneeling Runners Pose Quadriceps Stretch Sciatic Stretch	-Ask God why. -Tell God what you think. -Tell God what you feel. -Tell God what you want. -Thank God for what you have.	CARDIO I Loved You Then, 33 Miles Jesus Loves Me, Chris Tomlin Jesus Heals Your Heart, Third Day Love Is Not A Fight, Warren Barfield Love Never Fails, Brandon Heath Remind Me Who I Am, Jason Gray Unfailing Love, Chris Tomlin

DAY 4 SESSION 1

WARM UP STRETCHES Hold 10 - 20 seconds each	SPEAK LIFE I am good.	SONG LISTS FOR:
CARDIO	**PRAYER**	**STRETCHING** Offering, Third Day
Treadmill: 30–60 minutes Incline: 3 – 3.5 Speed: _____ Bike: 15 – 30 minutes Pedal as fast as you can. POST WORKOUT STRETCHES Hold 30 - 45 seconds each: Calf Stretch Hamstring Stretch IT Band Stretch Kneeling Runners Pose Quadriceps Stretch Sciatic Stretch	-Ask God questions. -Tell God what you think. -Tell God what you feel. -Tell God what you want. -Thank God for what you have. -Thank God for hearing your prayers.	**CARDIO** All The Broken Pieces, Matthew West By Your Side, Tenth Avenue North God Is Still God, Heather Williams He Is With Us, Love & The Outcome He Knows, Jeremy Camp Nothing Is Wasted, Jason Gray Promise Of A Lifetime, Kutless Strong Enough To Save, Tenth Avenue North

DAY 4 SESSION 2

WARM UP STRETCHES Hold 10 - 20 seconds each	SPEAK LIFE I am kind and caring.	SONG LISTS FOR:
CARDIO	**PRAYER**	**STRETCHING** Offering, Third Day
Treadmill: 30–60 minutes Incline: 3 – 3.5 Speed: _____ Elliptical: 15 minutes POST WORKOUT STRETCHES Hold 30 - 45 seconds each: Anterior Shoulder Stretch Calf Stretch Child's Pose Hamstring Stretch IT Band Stretch Neck / Trap Stretch Quadriceps Stretch Sciatic Stretch	-Ask God questions. -Tell God what you think. -Tell God what you feel. -Tell God what you want. -Thank God for what you have. -Thank God for hearing your prayers.	**CARDIO** All The Broken Pieces, Matthew West By Your Side, Tenth Avenue North God Is Still God, Heather Williams He Is With Us, Love & The Outcome He Knows, Jeremy Camp Nothing Is Wasted, Jason Gray Promise Of A Lifetime, Kutless Strong Enough To Save, Tenth Avenue North

DAY 5 SESSION 1

WARM UP STRETCHES	SPEAK LIFE	SONG LISTS FOR:
Hold 10 - 20 seconds each	I am blessed to be a blessing.	
		STRETCHING
CARDIO	**PRAYER**	Offering, Third Day
Treadmill: 30–60 minutes	-Ask God questions.	**CARDIO**
Incline: 4 – 4.5	-Tell God what you	All The Broken Pieces, Matthew
Speed: _____	think.	West
	-Tell God what you feel.	By Your Side, Tenth Avenue
Bike: 15 – 30 minutes	-Tell God what you want.	North
Pedal as fast as you can.	-Thank God for what you	God Is Still God, Heather
	have.	Williams
POST WORKOUT	-Thank God for hearing	He Is With Us, Love & The
STRETCHES	your prayers.	Outcome
Hold 30 - 45 seconds each:		He Knows, Jeremy Camp
		Nothing Is Wasted, Jason Gray
Calf Stretch		Promise Of A Lifetime, Kutless
Hamstring Stretch		Strong Enough To Save, Tenth
IT Band Stretch		Avenue North
Kneeling Runners Pose		
Quadriceps Stretch		
Sciatic Stretch		

DAY 5 SESSION 2

WARM UP STRETCHES	SPEAK LIFE	SONG LISTS FOR:
Hold 10 - 20 seconds each	I am getting through this.	
		STRETCHING
		Offering, Third Day
CARDIO	**PRAYER**	
Treadmill: 30–60 minutes	-Ask God questions.	**CARDIO**
Incline: 4 – 4.5	-Tell God what you	All The Broken Pieces, Matthew
Speed: _____	think.	West
	-Tell God what you feel.	Be Still, Story Side B
Bike: 15 – 30 minutes	-Tell God what you want.	He Knows My Name, Francesca
Pedal as fast as you can.	-Thank God for what you	Battistelli
	have.	Live Like That, Sidewalk
POST WORKOUT	-Thank God for hearing	Prophets Remind Me Who I
STRETCHES	your prayers.	Am, Jason Gray
Hold 30 - 45 seconds each:		Sea of Faces, Kutless
		You Are More, Tenth Avenue
Calf Stretch		North
Hamstring Stretch		
IT Band Stretch		
Kneeling Runners Pose		
Quadriceps Stretch		
Sciatic Stretch		

DAY 6 SESSION 1

WARM UP STRETCHES Hold 10 - 20 seconds each	SPEAK LIFE I am strong and able.	SONG LISTS FOR:
		STRETCHING
CARDIO	**PRAYER**	Offering, Third Day
Treadmill: 30–60 minutes	-Ask God questions.	CARDIO
Incline: 4 – 4.5	-Tell God what you	All The Broken Pieces,
Speed: _____	think.	Matthew West
Increase speed by 0 .5	-Tell God what you feel.	Be Still, Story Side B
	-Tell God what you	He Knows My Name,
Bike: 15 – 30 minutes	want.	Francesca Battistelli
Pedal as fast as you can.	-Thank God for	Live Like That, Sidewalk
	what you	Prophets Remind Me Who I
POST WORKOUT	have.	Am, Jason Gray
STRETCHES	-Thank God for hearing	Sea of Faces, Kutless
Hold 30 - 45 seconds each:	your	You Are More, Tenth Avenue
	prayers.	North
Calf Stretch		
Hamstring Stretch		
IT Band Stretch		
Kneeling Runners Pose		
Quadriceps Stretch		
Sciatic Stretch		

DAY 6 SESSION 2

WARM UP STRETCHES Hold 10 - 20 seconds each	SPEAK LIFE I am fit and healthy.	SONG LISTS FOR:
		STRETCHING
		Offering, Third Day
CARDIO	**PRAYER**	
Treadmill: 30–45 minutes	-Ask God questions.	CARDIO
Incline: 4 – 4.5	-Tell God what you	All The Broken Pieces,
Speed: _____	think.	Matthew West
	-Tell God what you feel.	Be Still, Story Side B
Elliptical: 15 – 30 minutes	-Tell God what you	He Knows My Name,
	want.	Francesca Battistelli
POST WORKOUT	-Thank God for	Live Like That, Sidewalk
STRETCHES	what you	Prophets Remind Me Who I
Hold 30 - 45 seconds each:	have.	Am, Jason Gray
	-Thank God for hearing	Sea of Faces, Kutless
Calf Stretch	your	You Are More, Tenth Avenue
Hamstring Stretch	prayers.	North
IT Band Stretch		
Kneeling Runners Pose		
Quadriceps Stretch		
Sciatic Stretch		

DAY 7

REST DAY	SPEAK LIFE I am hardworking.	SONG LISTS FOR: Play entire song list on shuffle.
STRETCHES Hold 30 - 45 seconds each: Do ALL Stretches	PRAYER -Speak to God about what's on your heart.	

DAY 8

WARM UP STRETCHES Hold 10 - 20 seconds each	SPEAK LIFE I am going to make it.	SONG LISTS FOR:
  CARDIO	 PRAYER	**STRETCHING** For The Glory Of It All, David Crowder
Treadmill: 30–45 minutes Incline: 5 Speed: _____ *Increase speed by 0.5*	-Praise God. -Confess your sins. -Ask for forgiveness. -Tell God what you are thinking. -Pray for other people. -Thank God for listening to you.	**CARDIO** For Those Who Wait, Fireflight I Still Believe, Jeremy Camp Savior Please, Josh Wilson There Will Be A Day, Jeremy Camp What Faith Can Do, Kutless **LEGS** God Is Enough, Lecrae Protection, Future of Forestry Rebel, Lecrae This Is Your Life, Switchfoot Walk On Water, Lecrae
LEGS 3 Sets Each	Weight/Rep	
Hack Squat: Wide Stance Hip Abduction Hip Adduction Leg Press Prone Leg Curl Seated Leg Curl Seated Leg Extensions Standing Calf Raises	/8 /8 /8 /8 /8 /8 /8 25	**POST WORKOUT STRETCHES** Hold 30 - 45 seconds each: Calf Stretch Hamstring Stretch IT Band Stretch Kneeling Runners Pose Quadriceps Stretch Sciatic Stretch

DAY 9

WARM UP STRETCHES Hold 10 - 20 seconds each	SPEAK LIFE I am a child of the Most High God.	SONG LISTS FOR:
CARDIO	**PRAYER**	**STRETCHING** For The Glory Of It All, David Crowder
Treadmill: 15 minutes Incline: 5 Speed: _____ *Increase speed by 0.5*	-Praise God. -Confess your sins. -Ask for forgiveness. -Tell God your feelings. -Tell God your needs. -Pray for other people. -Ask God to give you what He wants to give to you. -Thank God for what you have.	**CARDIO** For Those Who Wait, Fireflight I Still Believe, Jeremy Camp Savior Please, Josh Wilson There Will Be A Day, Jeremy Camp What Faith Can Do, Kutless **BACK / CHEST** Can't Take The Pain, Third Day Close Your Eyes, Future of Forestry East To West, Casting Crowns I Can Feel You, Bethel Music & J. Jonson More Time, Needtobreathe Praise You In The Storm, Casting Crowns Strong Tower, Kutless The Hurt And The Healer, Mercy Me Trust In You, Jeremy Camp
BACK / CHEST 3 Sets Each	Weight/Rep	
Back/Delt Press Extension Chest Press: Wide Grip Chest Press: Incline Lat Pull Down Lat Pull Down Reverse Push Ups Seated Row Vertical Butterfly	/8 /8 /8 /8 /8 10 /8 /8	**POST WORKOUT STRETCHES** Hold 30 - 45 seconds each: Bridge Cat Pose Chest Expansion Child's Pose Pectoral Stretch Seated Spinal Twist

DAY 10

WARM UP Stretch: 10 - 20 seconds each	SPEAK LIFE I am more than a conqueror.	SONG LISTS FOR:
CARDIO	**PRAYER**	**STRETCHING** For The Glory Of It All, David Crowder
Treadmill: 15 - 30 minutes Incline: 5 – 5.5 Speed: _____ *Increase speed by 0.5*	-Praise God. -Confess your sins. -Ask for forgiveness. -Tell God your feelings. -Tell God your needs. -Pray for other people. -Ask God to give you what He wants to give to you. -Thank God for what you have.	**CARDIO** For Those Who Wait, Fireflight I Still Believe, Jeremy Camp Savior Please, Josh Wilson There Will Be A Day, Jeremy Camp What Faith Can Do, Kutless **ARMS / SHOULDERS** Can't Take The Pain, Third Day Close Your Eyes, Future of Forestry East To West, Casting Crowns I Can Feel You, Bethel Music & J. Jonson More Time, Needtobreathe Praise You In The Storm, Casting Crowns Strong Tower, Kutless The Hurt And The Healer, Mercy Me Trust In You, Jeremy Camp
ARMS / SHOULDERS 3 Sets Each	Weight/Rep	
Bicep Curl Machine Deltoid Machine Dumbbell Rows Lat Pull Down Lat Pull Down Reverse Push Ups Triceps Dip Triceps Extension Machine	/8 /8 /8 /8 /8 10 10 /8	**POST WORKOUT STRETCHES** Hold 30 - 45 seconds each: Anterior Shoulder Stretch Bridge Cat Pose Chest Expansion Child's Pose Pectoral Stretch Tricep Stretch

DAY 11

WARM UP STRETCHES Hold 10 - 20 seconds each	SPEAK LIFE I am fearless.	SONG LISTS FOR:
CARDIO	**PRAYER**	**STRETCHING** For The Glory Of It All, David Crowder
Treadmill: 15 - 30 minutes Incline: 5 – 5.5 Speed: _____ *Increase speed by 0.5* Elliptical: 15 minutes	-Praise God. -Confess your sins. -Ask for forgiveness. -Ask for discernment. -Ask for wisdom. -Ask for guidance. -Ask for patience. -Tell God your feelings. -Tell God your needs. -Pray for other people. -Ask God to give you what He wants to give to you. -Thank God for what you have.	**CARDIO** Alive, Avalon Change In The Making, Addison Road Get Back Up, Toby Mac Glorious Day, Casting Crown I Will Rise, Chris Tomlison Speak Life, Toby Mac The Light In Me, Brandon Heath Walk On Water, Britt Nicole While I'm Waiting, John Waller **ABS / GLUTES** Can't Take The Pain, Third Day Close Your Eyes, Future of Forestry East To West, Casting Crowns I Can Feel You, Bethel Music & J. Jonson More Time, Needtobreathe Praise You In The Storm, Casting Crowns Strong Tower, Kutless The Hurt And The Healer, Mercy Me Trust In You, Jeremy Camp
ABS / GLUTES 4 Sets Each	Weight/Rep	
Abdominal Machine	/25	
Crunches	25	
Dead Lift	/8	**POST WORKOUT STRETCHES** Hold 30 - 45 seconds each:
Flutter Kicks	/8	
Good Mornings	/8	
Hamstring Curl	/8	Bridge
Leg Kickbacks	/8 each leg	Cat Pose
Plank	20 - 30 seconds	Child's Pose
Sit Ups	25	Sciatic Stretch
Sumo Squats with Dumbbell	/25	Seated Spinal Twist
V-Ups	25	

DAY 12

WARM UP STRETCHES Hold 10 - 20 seconds each	SPEAK LIFE I am smart and talented.	SONG LISTS FOR:
CARDIO	**PRAYER**	**STRETCHING** What Do You Know of Holy, Addison Road
Treadmill: 15 minutes Incline: 5 – 5.5 Speed: _____ *Increase speed by 0.5* Bike: 15 minutes Pedal as fast as you can. Elliptical: 15 minutes Stair Master: 15 minutes	-Thank God for what you have. -Confess your sins. -Ask for forgiveness. -Ask for peace. -Ask for your physical needs.	**CARDIO** For Those Who Wait, Fireflight I Still Believe, Jeremy Camp Savior Please, Josh Wilson There Will Be A Day, Jeremy Camp What Faith Can Do, Kutless **ARMS / SHOULDERS** Can't Take The Pain, Third Day Close Your Eyes, Future of Forestry East To West, Casting Crowns I Can Feel You, Bethel Music & J. Jonson More Time, Needtobreathe Praise You In The Storm, Casting Crowns Strong Tower, Kutless The Hurt And The Healer, Mercy Me Trust In You, Jeremy Camp
ARMS / SHOULDERS 3 Sets Each	Weight/Rep	
Bicep Curl Machine Deltoid Machine Dumbbell Rows Lat Pull Down Lat Pull Down Reverse Push Ups Triceps Dip Triceps Extension Machine	/8 /8 /8 /8 /8 10 10 /8	**POST WORKOUT** **STRETCHES** Hold 30 - 45 seconds each: Calf Stretch Hamstring Stretch IT Band Stretch Kneeling Runners Pose Quadriceps Stretch Sciatic Stretch Tricep Stretch

DAY 13

WARM UP STRETCHES Hold 10 - 20 seconds each	SPEAK LIFE I am likeable.	SONG LISTS FOR:
CARDIO	**PRAYER**	**STRETCHING** What Do You Know of Holy, Addison Road
Run / Walk Outside 45 – 75 minutes	-Speak to God about what's on your heart. -Thank God for a new day. -Thank God for His forgiveness. -Thank God for His love. -Thank God for His mercy. -Thank God for His grace.	**POST WORKOUT STRETCHES** Hold 30 - 45 seconds each: Do ALL Stretches

DAY 14

REST DAY	SPEAK LIFE I am funny.	SONG LISTS FOR: Play entire song list on shuffle.
STRETCHES Hold 30 - 45 seconds each: Do ALL Stretches	**PRAYER** -Speak to God about what's on your heart.	

DAY 15

WARM UP STRETCHES Hold 10 - 20 seconds each	SPEAK LIFE I can forgive and I am forgiven.	SONG LISTS FOR:
		STRETCHING What Do You Know of Holy
CARDIO	**PRAYER**	Addison Road
Treadmill: 15 minutes Incline: 5.5 - 6 Speed: _____ *Increase speed by 0.5*	-Praise God. -Confess your sins. -Ask for forgiveness. -Tell God what you are thinking. -Pray for other people. -Thank God for listening to you. -Thank God for what you have.	**CARDIO** Courageous, Casting Crowns This Is Your Life, Switchfoot Word of God Speak, Mercy Me Worn, Tenth Avenue North **LEGS** All Around Me, Flyleaf Fighter, Manafest God Is Enough, Lecrae God's Not Dead, Newsboys Go Hard, Lecrae Made To Love, Toby Mac Move, Mercy Me Movin, Group 1 Crew Overcomer, Mandisa Protection, Future of Forestry Rebel, Lecrae Walk On Water, Lecrae
LEGS 4 Sets Each	Weight/Rep	
Hack Squat: Wide Stance Hip Abduction Hip Adduction Leg Press Lunges: Dumbbell Prone Leg Curl Seated Leg Curl Seated Leg Extensions Standing Calf Raises	/8 /8 /8 /8 /10 each leg /8 /8 /8 25	**POST WORKOUT STRETCHES** Hold 30 - 45 seconds each: Calf Stretch Hamstring Stretch IT Band Stretch Kneeling Runners Pose Quadriceps Stretch Sciatic Stretch

DAY 16

WARM UP STRETCHES	SPEAK LIFE	SONG LISTS FOR:
Hold 10 - 20 seconds each	God loves me and cares about me.	
		STRETCHING
		What Do You Know of Holy
CARDIO	**PRAYER**	Addison Road
Treadmill: 8 minutes	-Praise God.	**CARDIO**
Incline: 6	-Confess your sins.	All of Me, Matt Hammitt
Speed: _____	-Ask God to show you	Beautiful Things, Gungor
Increase speed by 0.5	what	Courageous, Casting Crowns
	you need to confess.	Everything, Lifehouse
Bike: 12 minutes	-Ask for forgiveness.	Micah 6:8, Charlie Hall
Pedal as fast as you can.	-Tell God your secrets.	Never Letting Go, Nickelback
	-Ask God for the	One Thing Remains, Soul
Elliptical: 15 minutes	things you	Survivor
Stair Master: 10 minutes	want.	So Small, Carrie Underwood
	-Ask to fulfill God's	This Is Your Life, Switchfoot
	will for	Words I Would Say, Sidewalk
	your life.	Prophets
	-Ask to have your heart	
	aligned with His.	**BACK & ABS**
	-Thank God for the	Home, Phillip Phillips
	people in	If Today Was Your Last Day,
	your life.	Nickelback
	-Pray for other people.	I'm Wide Awake, Katy Perry
	-Thank God for	Joy Unspeakable, Mandisa
	listening to	Let It Fade, Jeremy Camp
	you.	Let It Roll, Group 1 Crew
	-Thank God for what you have.	
BACK 3 Sets Each	Weight/Rep	
Back / Delt Press Ext	/10	
Bent Over Barbell Row	/10	
Lat Pull Down Reverse	/10	
Pull Ups: With(out) asst	/10	
Seated Row	/10	
ABS 4 Sets Each	Weight/Rep	
Abdominal Machine	/25	
Crunches	25	**POST WORKOUT**
Flutter Kicks	/25 each leg	**STRETCHES**
Good Mornings	/25	Hold 30 - 45 seconds each:
Plank	20 - 30 seconds	
Sit Ups	25	Do ALL Stretches
V-Ups	25	

DAY 17

WARM UP STRETCHES	SPEAK LIFE	SONG LISTS FOR:
Hold 10 - 20 seconds each	I am loyal and trustworthy.	
		STRETCHING
		What Do You Know of Holy, Addison Road
CARDIO	**PRAYER**	**CARDIO**
Treadmill: 10 minutes	-Tell God how good He	Busted Heart, For King &
Incline: 6 - 7	is.	Country
Speed: _____	-Ask God to show you	Courageous, Casting Crowns
Increase speed by 0.5	what you need to	Everything Falls, Fee
	confess.	Lessons Learned, Carrie
Bike: 15 minutes	-Ask for forgiveness.	Underwood
Pedal as fast as you can.	-Tell God your secrets.	Life Ain't Always Beautiful, Gary
	-Ask God to help you	Allan
Elliptical: 15 minutes	forgive those who	Losing, Tenth Avenue North
Stair Master: 15 minutes	have hurt you.	Safe, Phil Wickham
	-Thank God for the	Sound Of Your Voice, Third Day
	lessons you are	Word Of God Speak, Mercy Me
	learning.	
	-Ask to fulfill God's will	**CHEST**
	for your life.	Home, Phillip Phillips
	-Pray for other people.	If Today Was Your Last Day,
	-Thank God for	Nickelback
	changing you.	I'm Wide Awake, Katy Perry
	-Thank God for who He	Joy Unspeakable, Mandisa
	is.	Let It Fade, Jeremy Camp
		Let It Roll, Group 1 Crew
CHEST 3 Sets Each	Weight/Rep	
Cable Cross Over	/10	
Chest Press	/10	
Chest Press Incline	/10	
Dumbbell Fly	/10	
Seated Row	/10	
Vertical Butterfly		
ABS 4 Sets Each	Weight/Rep	
Crunches	25	
Flutter Kicks	25 each leg	**POST WORKOUT STRETCHES**
Plank	30 - 40 seconds	Hold 30 - 45 seconds each:
Roman Twist	20 each side	
Sit Ups	25	Child's Pose
V-Ups	25	Chest Expansion
		Pectoral Stretch
		Neck / Trap Stretch

DAY 18

WARM UP STRETCHES	SPEAK LIFE	SONG LISTS FOR:
Hold 10 - 20 seconds each	I am faithful.	
CARDIO	**PRAYER**	**STRETCHING**
		Healing Oil, Kim Walker-Smith
Treadmill: 10 minutes	-Thank God for today.	**CARDIO**
Incline: 7 – 7.5	-Ask God to forgive you.	Busted Heart, For King &
Speed: _____	-Tell God your thoughts.	Country
	-Tell God you want His	Courageous, Casting Crowns
Bike: 15 minutes	will for	Everything Falls, Fee
Pedal as fast as you can.	your life.	Lessons Learned, Carrie
	-Ask God to bless you	Underwood Life Ain't Always
Elliptical: 15 minutes	so you	Beautiful, Gary Allan
Stair Master: 15 minutes	can bless others.	Losing, Tenth Avenue North
	-Pray for other people.	Safe, Phil Wickham
	-Thank God for	Sound Of Your Voice, Third Day
	everything you	Word Of God Speak, Mercy Me
	have.	**ARMS**
		Home, Phillip Phillips
		If Today Was Your Last Day, Nickelback
		I'm Wide Awake, Katy Perry
		Joy Unspeakable, Mandisa
		Let It Fade, Jeremy Camp
		Let It Roll, Group 1 Crew
ARMS 4 Sets Each	Weight/Rep	
Dumbbell Bicep Curl	/10	
Dumbbell Hammer	/10	
Curl Dumbbell Triceps	/10	
Extension	/10	
Rope Extension		
ABS 4 Sets Each	Weight/Rep	
Crunches	25	
Flutter Kicks	25 each leg	**POST WORKOUT**
Plank	40 - 50 seconds	**STRETCHES**
Push Ups	12	Hold 30 - 45 seconds each:
Roman Twist	20 each side	
Sit Ups	25	Child's Pose
V-Ups	25	Chest Expansion
		Pectoral Stretch
		Neck / Trap Stretch

DAY 19

WARM UP STRETCHES Hold 10 - 20 seconds each	SPEAK LIFE I am desirable.	SONG LISTS FOR:
CARDIO	PRAYER	**STRETCHING** Healing Oil, Kim Walker-Smith
Treadmill: 8 minutes Incline: 7.5 – 8 Speed: _____ Bike: 10 minutes Pedal as fast as you can. Elliptical: 12 minutes Stair Master: 10 minutes	-Thank God for today. -Ask God to forgive you. -Ask God to make you a fast learner. -Ask God to help you forgive yourself. -Ask God to open and close all the doors that need to be opened or closed to lead to your destiny. -Pray for other people. -Thank God for what you have.	**CARDIO** Forgiveness, Toby Mac Losing, Tenth Avenue North 7 x 70, Chris August **SHOULDERS & ABS** Alive, Hillsong Young & Free Better Than I Used To Be, Tim McGraw I Believe, Seventh Day Slumber Invincible, Kelly Clarkson I Will Follow, Chris Tomlin Learning To Be The Light, New World Son Lord I'm Ready Now, Plumb
SHOULDERS 4 Sets Each	Weight/Rep	
Dumbbell Front Raise	/10	
Dumbbell Lateral Raise	/10	
Dumbbell Shoulder Raise	/10	
Pull Up Machine	/10	
Push Ups	15	
ABS 4 Sets Each	Weight/Rep	
Crunches	25	
Flutter Kicks	25 each leg	**POST WORKOUT**
Plank	40 - 50 seconds	**STRETCHES**
Roman Twist	20 each side	Hold 30 - 45 seconds each:
Sit Ups	25	
V-Ups	25	Do ALL stretches.

DAY 20

WARM UP STRETCHES Hold 10 - 20 seconds each	SPEAK LIFE I am compassionate.	SONG LISTS FOR:
CARDIO	**PRAYER**	**STRETCHING** Forgiveness, Matthew West
Run / Walk Outside 45 – 75 minutes **POST WORKOUT STRETCHES** Hold 30 - 45 seconds each: Do ALL Stretches	-Give God praise. -Speak to God about what's and who is on your heart. -Ask God to show you how He sees other people. -Ask for a compassionate heart. -Ask for the words to speak. -Thank God everything.	**CARDIO** Beautiful, Christina Aguilera Everything Good, The Afters Gold, Britt Nicole Hall Of Fame, The Script ft. Will I Am Perfect, Pink Press On, Mandisa Stronger, Kelly Clarkson Try, Pink Who Says, Selena Gomez Who You Are, Jessie J

DAY 21

REST DAY	SPEAK LIFE I am interesting and people like me.	SONG LISTS FOR: Play entire song list on shuffle.
STRETCHES Hold 30 - 45 seconds each: Do ALL Stretches	**PRAYER** -Speak to God about what's on your heart. -Ask God to transform your life. -Give Him praises for everything.	

DAY 22

WARM UP STRETCHES Hold 10 - 20 seconds each	SPEAK LIFE I can do all things through Christ.	SONG LISTS FOR:
CARDIO	**PRAYER**	**STRETCHING** Mighty Breath Of God, Jesus Culture
Treadmill: 5 minutes Incline: 8 – 8.5 Speed: _____ Bike: 5 minutes Pedal as fast as you can. Elliptical: 5 minutes Stair Master: 5 minutes	-Give God honor. -Confess your sins. -Ask God for forgiveness. -Thank God for His forgiveness. -Tell God to use you for His glory. -Thank Him because He will. -Ask God to help you forgive yourself. -Ask God to heal your heart, mind and spirit. -Thank God for His faithfulness.	**CARDIO** Came To My Rescue, Hillsong United Forgiveness, Matthew West Losing, Tenth Avenue North Speak Life, Toby Mac 7 x 70, Chris August **GLUTES** Alive, Hillsong Young & Free Better Than I Used To Be, Tim McGraw I Believe, Seventh Day Slumber Invincible, Kelly Clarkson I Will Follow, Chris Tomlin Learning To Be The Light, New World Son Lord I'm Ready Now, Plumb Whatever You're Doing, Sanctus Real
GLUTES 5 Sets Each	Weight/Rep	
Deadlift Dumbbell Squats Dumbbell Sumo Squats Leg Kickbacks	/12 /12 /12 12 each leg	**POST WORKOUT** **STRETCHES** Hold 30 - 45 seconds each: Do ALL stretches.

DAY 23

WARM UP STRETCHES Hold 10 - 20 seconds each	SPEAK LIFE God is taking care of all of my needs.	SONG LISTS FOR:
		STRETCHING The Heart Of Worship, Passion Worship Band
CARDIO	**PRAYER**	
Treadmill: 5 minutes	-Give God honor.	**HIIT**
Incline: 8.5 – 9	-Confess your sins.	Dear X, Disciple
Speed: _____	-Ask God for forgiveness.	Forever Reign, Passion Worship
	-Thank God for His forgiveness.	Band Forgiven, Sanctus Real
Bike: 5 minutes	-Tell God to use you for His	Give Me Your Eyes, Brandon
Pedal as fast as you can.	glory.	Heath
	-Thank Him because He will.	I Refuse, Josh Wilson
Elliptical: 5 minutes	-Thank God for what you are	King Of Glory, Third Day
Stair Master: 5 minutes	going through.	Ready, Third Day
	-Ask for more faith.	Take My Life, Jeremy Camp
	-Thank God for His	The Lost Get Found, Britt Nicole
	faithfulness.	Unbreakable, Fireflight
		7x70, Chris August
HIIT 2 Sets Each High Intensity Interval Training	Weight/Rep	
ROUND 1		
Jump Rope	1 minute	
Lunges	15 each leg	
Jump Rope	1 minute	
Free Hand Jump Squat	20	
Jump Rope	1 minute	* If you don't have a jump rope
Rest/Break	45 seconds	you can do 1 minute of jumping
		jacks in place of the jump rope*
ROUND 2		
Jump Rope	1 minute	
Sit Ups	20	
Burpee with a Jump	10	
Push Ups	10	
High Knees	50 (25 each knee)	**POST WORKOUT**
Jump Rope	1 minute	**STRETCHES**
Rest/Break	30 seconds	Hold 30 - 45 seconds each:
ROUND 3		Do ALL stretches.
Jumping Jacks	40	
Roman Twist	20 (10 each side)	
Mountain Climbers	50 (25 each leg)	
Air Squats	50	
Jumping Jacks	40	
Side Plank	30 seconds each side	
Jumping Jacks	40	

DAY 24

WARM UP STRETCHES Hold 10 - 20 seconds each	SPEAK LIFE I am thankful.	SONG LISTS FOR:
CARDIO	**PRAYER**	**STRETCHING** Show Me Your Glory, Jesus Culture
Treadmill: 5 minutes Incline: 9 Speed: _____ Bike: 5 minutes Pedal as fast as you can. Elliptical: 5 minutes Stair Master: 5 minutes	-Give God honor. -Confess your sins. -Ask God for forgiveness. -Ask God to bring you the people you need. -Ask God to remove the people in your life that you don't need. -Thank God for what you are going through. -Ask for more faith. -Thank God for His faithfulness.	**PLYOMETRICS** Dear X, Disciple Forever Reign, Passion Worship Band Forgiven, Sanctus Real Give Me Your Eyes, Brandon Heath I Refuse, Josh Wilson King Of Glory, Third Day Ready, Third Day Take My Life, Jeremy Camp The Lost Get Found, Britt Nicole Unbreakable, Fireflight 7x70, Chris August
PLYOMETRICS 3 Sets Each	Weight/Rep	
Alternating High Knee	40 (20 each leg)	**POST WORKOUT STRETCHES** Hold 30 - 45 seconds each: Do ALL stretches.
Box Jumps	20	
Double Leg Butt Kick	15	
High Knees	50 (25 each leg)	
Jumping Lunges	40 (20 each leg)	
Jump Squats	20	
Jumping Jacks	40	
Lateral Lunges	40 (20 each leg)	
Plie Jump Squat	20	
Side to Side Box Shuffle	40 (20 each side)	
Split Squat Jumps	50 (25 each leg)	
30 second rest between sets		

DAY 25

WARM UP STRETCHES	SPEAK LIFE	SONG LISTS FOR:
Hold 10 - 20 seconds each	I am an overcomer.	
		STRETCHING
CARDIO	**PRAYER**	Fill Me Up, Jesus Culture
Treadmill: 5 minutes	Sing the words of the song as	**CARDIO & FULL**
Incline: 9	your prayer today.	**BODY WORKOUT**
Speed: _____		Shuffle Entire Song List
Increase Speed by 0.5		
ARMS / SHOULDERS	Weight/Reps	
2 Sets		
Bicep Curl (straight bar)	/10	
Front Raise (straight bar)	/10	
Pull Ups	/10	
Shoulder Press (straight bar)	/10	
Skull Crusher (straight bar)	/10	
ABS / GLUTES 2 Sets	Weight/Reps	
Crunches	25	
Deadlifts	/10	
Donkey Kicks	50 (25 each leg)	
Flutter Kicks	50 (25 each leg)	
In & Outs	25	
Plank	60 seconds	
Scissors	25	
V-Ups	25	
BACK / CHEST 2 Sets	Weight/Reps	
Bent Over Rows	/10	
(straight bar)	/10	
Chest Press	/10	
Incline Chest Press	/10	
(straight bar)	10	
Lat Pull Down	10	
Push Ups	10	
Pull Ups	10	
LEGS 2 Sets	Weight/Reps	
Front Squats (straight bar)	/10	
Lateral Lunges	/10 each leg	**POST WORKOUT**
Lunges	/10 each leg	**STRETCHES**
Squats (straight bar)	/10	Hold 30 - 45 seconds
Walking Lunges	/10	each:
(straight bar)	/10	
		Do ALL stretches

DAY 26

WARM UP STRETCHES Hold 10 - 20 seconds each	SPEAK LIFE I am humble.	SONG LISTS FOR:
CARDIO	PRAYER	STRETCHING Freedom Reign, Jesus Culture
Treadmill: 10 minutes Incline: 10 Speed: _____	-Praise God. -Confess your sins. -Ask for forgiveness. -Ask God to show you things you do not know. -Ask God for discernment. -Ask God for wisdom. -Ask God to give and reveal your spiritual gifts. -Thank God for transforming you. -Thank God for His will.	CARDIO & FULL BODY WORKOUT Even When, Jeremy Camp Grace Like Rain, Todd Agnew I Feel So Alive, Capital Kings If Today Was Your Last Day, Nickelback I'm Wide Awake, Katy Perry Joy Unspeakable, Mandisa Let It Fade, Jeremy Camp Take It All, Third Day
WORKOUT 4 Sets	Weight/Reps	
Air Squats Alternating Side Plank Crunches Jumping Jacks Leg Raises Push Ups Burpees High Knees Jump Squats Sit Ups Jump Rope	50 30 seconds each side 25 50 50 (25 each leg) 20 25 50 (25 each knee) 25 25 2 minutes	POST WORKOUT STRETCHES Hold 30 - 45 seconds each: Do ALL stretches

DAY 27

WARM UP STRETCHES Hold 10 - 20 seconds each	SPEAK LIFE I have a purpose.	SONG LISTS FOR:
CARDIO	**PRAYER**	**STRETCHING** Mighty Breath Of God, Jesus Culture
Treadmill: 5 minutes Incline: 10.5 Speed: _____	-Thank you God for loving me and for knowing what is best for me. You are the great, I am. Thank You for your will for my life and that I will fulfill it. Thank You for forgiving me and for giving me a forgiving heart. Thank You for not leaving me and for always making a way for me. Thank You for hearing my prayers.	**CARDIO** Dear X, Disciple Forever Reign, Passion Worship Band Forgiven, Sanctus Real Give Me Your Eyes, Brandon Heath I Refuse, Josh Wilson King Of Glory, Third Day Ready, Third Day Take My Life, Jeremy Camp The Lost Get Found, Britt Nicole Unbreakable, Fireflight 7x70, Chris August **HIIT** Shuffle Entire Song List.
HIIT 2 Sets Each High Intensity Interval Training	Weight/Rep	
ROUND 1 Jump Rope 1 Hand Kettle Bell Swing Jump Rope Plank Jump Rope Rest/Break	2 minutes 40 (20 each hand) 2 minutes 1 minute 2 minutes 45 seconds	* If you don't have a jump rope you can do 2 minutes of jumping jacks in place of the jump rope*
ROUND 2 Box Jump Speed Skater 2 Hand Kettle Bell Swing Medicine Ball Overhead Throw High Knees Hold Squat / Wall Sit Rest/Break	20 1 minute 40 20 50 (25 each knee) 1 minute 30 seconds 25	**POST WORKOUT STRETCHES** Hold 30 - 45 seconds each: Do ALL stretches.
ROUND 3 Medicine Ball Slam Roman Twist Jog In Place Air Squats Jumping Jacks Side Plank Jumping Jacks Sit Ups	20 (10 each side) 1 minute 50 40 30 seconds each side 40 25	

DAY 28

WARM UP STRETCHES Hold 10 - 20 seconds each	SPEAK LIFE I am forgiven and I have been redeemed.	SONG LISTS FOR:
WORKOUT Walk Outside for 1 Hour Listening to Song List and Throughout the Day. **POST WORKOUT STRETCHES** Hold 30 - 45 seconds each: Do ALL Stretches	**PRAYER** Thank You God for who You are. Please forgive me of my sins. Thank you for turning my pain to joy. Thank you for telling me who I am to you. Thank you that I matter to you. Thank you for your blessings. Thank You for healing me and for turning my pain into joy. Thank You for fighting for me. Thank You, God for all things in my life. Thank You for changing me, my life, my mind, my point of view, my relationship with You.	**STRETCHES** Beautiful, Fellowship Creative **WALK** Blessed, Martina McBride Fight Song, Rachel Platten How You Live, Point Of Grace I Hope You Dance, LeeAnn Womack Just Stand Up, Carrie Underwood Little Wonders, Rob Thomas Overcomer, Mandisa Roar, Katy Perry Say, John Mayer Stronger, Mandisa Survivor, Destiny's Child Titanium, David Guetta ft. Sia

DAY 29

WARM UP STRETCHES Hold 10 - 20 seconds each	SPEAK LIFE I am hopeful.	SONG LISTS FOR:
CARDIO	**PRAYER**	**STRETCHING** Fill Me Up, Jesus Culture
Treadmill: 10 minutes Incline: 10 Speed: _____		**CARDIO** Fight Song, Rachel Platten
Bike: 10 minutes Pedal as fast as you can.		Just Stand Up, Carrie Underwood Overcomer, Mandisa Roar, Katy Perry
Elliptical: 10 minutes Stair Master: 5 minutes		Stronger, Mandisa Survivor, Destiny's Child Titanium, David Guetta ft. Sia
		ARMS Repeat Cardio Song List
ARMS 4 Sets	Weight/Rep	
Bicep Curl	/12	
Cable Curl	/12	
Cable Pull-Down	/12	**POST WORKOUT**
Hammer Curl	/12	**STRETCHES**
Incline Curl	/12	Hold 30 - 45 seconds
Kickback	/12	each:
Overhead Dumbbell Ext	/12	
Skullcrusher	/12	Child's Pose
Tricep Push-Down	/12	Chest Expansion Pectoral Stretch Neck / Trap Stretch

DAY 30

WARM UP STRETCHES Hold 10 - 20 seconds each	SPEAK LIFE God has transformed my heart, my mind, my soul, and my life.	SONG LISTS FOR:
WORKOUT	**PRAYER**	**STRETCHING** Beautiful, Fellowship Creative
Run / Walk Outside 45 – 75 minutes **POST WORKOUT STRETCHES** Hold 30 - 45 seconds each: Do ALL Stretches	Read below.	**WORKOUT** Play entire song list on shuffle.

Day 30 Prayer:

Father God,

Thank you for carrying me through. Thank you for being with me, and helping me and for making a way for me. Thank you for not ever leaving me. I ask for your forgiveness for my sins and for making me right before you. Thank you for changing and transforming my heart and my life. Thank you for your love for me. Thank you for showing me who I am to you and for helping me to love and forgive others and myself. I want you to come into my heart and to lead my life and be the center of my every thing. Help me to become everything you created me to be. May your will be done in my life. Thank you that it will be. In Jesus' name. Amen.

Chapter 12

30 DAY GENERAL MEAL PLAN

GUIDELINES

- Always see a doctor before starting this meal plan or any other meal plan. *Note: All supplements are recommendations/suggestions, consult your doctor prior to taking or using any of them.*

- Eat 6 meals a day, every 2-3hrs. Do NOT eat an hour before bedtime.

- Eat food for meal 1 within 30 minutes of waking up. Do NOT drink coffee, a shake or a smoothie as your breakfast unless it is a shake with protein in it.

- Read the labels! Do NOT eat packaged, processed, boxed, or canned foods that have sugar grams over 10. Keep the grams of sugar under 10g.

- Eat carbs and foods low in sugar during breakfast and lunch. No carbs with dinner. (For allowed carbs see list).

- Take your vitamins and supplements.

- Do 60 - 90 minutes of cardio per day. (You can break it up if you need to: e.g. 60 in the morning, 30 at night or 3 – 30 minute sessions etc.).

- Get at least 8 hours of sleep at night. Take naps as needed throughout the day.

- NO Sweets: cake, soda, Kool-Aid, ice cream, brownies, muffins, cupcakes, pastries, cookies Etc.

- NO Alcohol (1 glass of red wine per week is permitted - optional)

- NO Sugar, Fried Foods, Dairy, Starches (see allowed carb list for allowed starches).

- Drink 1 gallon of water per day.

<u>MEALS</u>

Meal 1:
- Carb, Protein, Vegetable, and Supplements (Fish Oil, Multi Vitamin)
- Drink at least 16oz of water.
- Drink hot Green, White, or Oolong Tea or black coffee. (or you can purchase the Herbalife Fat Burner Tea/ Metabolism Booster Tea from my website – optional)

Meal 2:
- Protein Shake and Supplements (Vitamin C & Vitamin D). If still hungry, eat a green vegetable with 1 carb, or drink a green juice.
- Drink at least 24oz of water.

Meal 3:
- Carb, Protein, Vegetable, and Supplements (Vitamin E, Iron)
- Drink at least 16oz of water.
- Drink hot Green, White, or Oolong Tea.

Meal 4:
- Protein Shake and Supplements (CoQ10 & CLA (conjugated linoleic acid))
- Drink at least 24oz of water.

Meal 5:
- Protein and a Vegetable. (Brown Seaweed & Black Licorice)
- Drink at least 16oz of water.
- Drink Decaffeinated Green Tea.

Meal 6:
- Protein Shake and 32oz of water

Meal Examples

Example 1

Meal 1: 2-3 Egg Whites (1 yolk if 3 eggs) cooked in one of the oils with at least 2 handfuls of spinach and or kale. You can substitute egg whites with chicken, turkey or fish. Fruit is allowed.

Meal 2: Protein Shake mixed ONLY with water. If still hungry eat broccoli, celery sticks and a spoon of low fat, low sugar almond / peanut butter or cottage cheese. Fruit is allowed.

Meal 3: A salad with a lean meat, turkey, tuna, and or chicken breast. You can add nuts and or boiled eggs, dried fruits.

No cheese, except ¼ cup of cottage cheese. Allowed dressing: olive oil and or balsamic vinaigrette. Salt & pepper and/or Mrs. Dash or Flavor God seasonings.

Meal 4: Protein Shake mixed ONLY with water. No fruit. Green vegetables allowed if still hungry.

Meal 5: A Salad with a lean meat, turkey, tuna, chicken breast. You can add nuts and/or boiled eggs, dried fruits. No croutons, or dressing unless it is olive oil and/or balsamic vinaigrette. Salt & pepper and/or Mrs. Dash.

Meal 6: A lean meat, with lots of vegetables. Or you can eat Meal 1 again.

Example 2

Meal 1: 1 cup of steel cut oatmeal mixed with 1 scoop of protein powder. Add cinnamon and/or stevia if you would like or a small spoon of coconut oil. NO butter or milk. Almond or flax milk is okay. 2 egg whites, and 1 whole egg. ¼ of an avocado and spinach.

Meal 2: Protein shake add cinnamon if you like. If still hungry eat a vegetable or a protein bar (read sugar content, <10g) or some nuts. Fruit is allowed.

Meal 3: Lean meat with either ½ cup of brown rice, quinoa, or sweet potato and dark green vegetable. ½ cup of blueberries or strawberries.

Meal 4: Protein shake add cinnamon if you like. If still hungry eat a vegetable or ½ cup of honey dew or ½ a grapefruit. NO protein bar .

Meal 5: Lean meat and dark green vegetables.

Meal 6: A Salad with a lean meat, turkey, tuna, or chicken breast. You can add nuts and/or boiled eggs. No cheese, croutons, or dried fruit. Salad dressing allowed: olive oil and/or balsamic vinaigrette.

Example 3

Meal 1: Egg white omelet with ground turkey or turkey bacon (on the side). Add spinach, onions, tomatoes, cilantro, jalapenos. Avocados on the side. Fruit allowed.

Meal 2: Protein shake add cinnamon if you like. Add a berry or berries and a banana to it. (strawberry, blueberry, black berry, raspberry etc)

Meal 3: Lean meat with either brown rice, quinoa, sweet potato and dark green vegetables. ½ cup of berries.

Meal 4: Protein shake and a Green juice.

Meal 5: Lean meat and dark green vegetables. No carbs.

Meal 6: A Salad with a lean meat, turkey, tuna, chicken breast. You can add nuts and/or boiled eggs. No cheese, croutons, or dried fruits. Salad dressing allowed: olive oil and/or balsamic vinaigrette.

NOTES

- Dark Green Vegetables: asparagus, broccoli, spinach, celery, kale, cucumbers, zucchini.

- Bake, grill, boil, broil, sauté, or pan sear (do not fry) meats and vegetables.

- **NO** sugar. If you must sweeten something use cinnamon, agave, stevia, or raw honey.

- **Cooking oils** allowed: safflower, olive, coconut, walnut, or sesame.

- **Seasonings** allowed: Mrs. Dash – any flavor. Flavor God seasoning – any flavor. Cinnamon, Black Pepper, Sarachi Hot Sauce, Red Pepper Flakes, Cayenne Pepper, Mustard, Ground Brown Mustard, Tarragon.

- Eat these peppers with meals 1, 3, & 5 if you like: Jalapeno, or Habaneros. Add garlic, ginger, and onions to any meal.

- If you're desiring something sweet after meal 6. Freeze your protein shake and add cinnamon. It will make your brain think your eating ice cream.

- If you drink Oolong Tea you can add Stevia to it because it's a little bitter.

Supplements are optional. Speak to a doctor before taking any kinds of medicine or supplements See supplement list or visit my website: **alysiarieg.com** to see what I use or register **https://www.goherbalife.com/alysiarieg.**

Allowed Carbs	Proteins	Supplements
Quinoa	Chicken Breast	Vitamin C
Sweet Potatoes	Turkey	Vitamin E
Brown Rice	Fish	CLA (conjugated linoleic acid)

Seaweed	Shrimp	Brown Seaweed & Black Licorice
Prunes	Sardines	Iron
Raisins	Black Beans	Lysine
Blueberries	Lentils	Multi Vitamin
Watermelon	Kidney Beans	CoQ10
Grapefruit	Egg Whites	Fish Oil
Collard Greens	Vitamin D	

Green Vegetables	Add Ons or Sides (optional)
Broccoli	Cilantro
Cabbage	Onions
Kale	Avocado
Spinach	Pico de Gallo
Okra	Peppers
Asparagus	
Green Beans	

Green Juice
Juice in Juicer or Blend in Blender

Examples:
- Water, kale, spinach, cucumber, pineapple, grapes, pear, ginger, green apple.
- Mint, spinach, kale, banana, apple juice, spirulina, probiotic, ginger, aloe vera juice.
- Ginger, spinach, cucumber, pineapple juice, apple, lettuce, lemon, parsley, grape.
- Spinach, banana, pomegranate seeds, super green powder.
- Kale, spinach, spirulina, apple juice, kiwi, banana.
- Water, super green powder, apple, banana
- Juice with Prime Nutrition's Phytoform.

For other juices/smoothies see my Facebook page ALYSIA RIEG (athlete) under the album Juices-Smoothies.

See my website **alysiarieg.com** or email me at forsuchatimeasthisbook@gmail.com

Lastly, diet is 90% of weight loss. If you cheat, you're not cheating me, but yourself.

Use code ALYSIA20 at primenutrition.com to get a discount on the Phytoform if you choose to purchase it.

YOU EITHER WANT IT OR YOU DON'T!

Stretches

ANTERIOR SHOULDER STRETCH: Reach your arm across your body and hold it straight. With opposite hand, grasp the elbow that is across your body and pull it across your body towards your chest. Hold stretch. Remember to breathe. Repeat on other side.

BRIDGE: Lay on back, bending both knees with both feet flat on the ground. Feet should be about hip-width apart.

Bend elbows to 90 degrees so that hands are on the ground, fingertips pointed towards feet.

Then drive up through your heels and upper back lifting glutes up off the ground. Drive your hips up as high as possible, squeezing the glutes hard. Keep your belly button drawn in towards spine so back does not hyper extend.

Do not push backward off your heels. Make sure to drive straight up and knees aren't caving in.

Squeeze your glutes for 10 seconds at the top and lower all the way back down to the ground before repeating.

CALF STRETCH: Stand facing a wall. Extend your arms in front of you placing hands flat on the wall, keeping the elbows slightly bent. Keep both feet flat, step or slide one foot back behind you on floor, lengthening leg and press hands onto wall giving a gentle push. You should feel the stretch in the calf of the extended leg. To get a deeper stretch slowly lower heel of extended leg to the floor. Breathe deeply holding stretch for 10-30 seconds. Repeat with opposite leg.

CAT POSE: Start on your hands (fingers pointed forward with hands flat to ground) and knees in a "tabletop" position. Make sure your knees are directly below your hips and your wrists, elbows and shoulders are in line, perpendicular to the floor. Center your head in a neutral position, eyes looking at the floor.

On exhale, round spine toward the ceiling, making sure to keep shoulders and knees in position. Release your head toward floor, do not force chin to chest.

CHEST EXPANSION: Sit or stand up tall and bring your arms behind you, clasping one hand inside the other. Lift your chest and raise your arms slightly. Stretch is felt spread across chest.

CHILD'S POSE: Kneel on the floor. Touch your big toes together and sit on your heels, separate knees as wide as your hips. Arms stretched out in front of you on the ground.

Exhale laying torso down between your thighs. Broaden your sacrum across the back of pelvis narrowing hip points toward the navel, so that they nestle down onto the inner thighs. Lengthen your tailbone away from the back of the pelvis while lifting the base of skull away from the back of neck.

Bring hands on the floor along side torso, palms up, and release the fronts of your shoulders toward the floor.

HAMSTRING STRETCH: Lie on your back with one leg extended and back straight. Keep hips leveled to the ground keeping lower back down towards the floor. Bend either knee towards chest, keeping other leg extended on the floor. Straighten the knee that is towards chest extending leg vertically above you. Then grab the back of the vertical leg with both hands. Pull your vertical leg towards you gently keeping hips on the floor. Hold stretch for10-30 seconds. Remember to breathe. Repeat with opposite leg. If you are unable to extend the leg, you may keep the knee bent pulling behind your leg near hamstring and pull gently towards your chest, alternating with the other leg after a 10-30 second hold.

ILLOTIBIAL (IT) BAND STRETCH: With one side of your body next to a wall, stand tall with your hand pressed onto wall and body arm length away. Cross one leg in front of the other leg (leg closest to the wall) and place your opposite hand on your hip, shoulders relaxed, feet flat on the floor. Breathing slowly and deeply, steadily push your hip towards the wall, bending elbow slightly. Keep the foot closest to the wall flat on the floor, both legs straight, and your back straight. Hold the stretch for 10-30 seconds. Switch and repeat on opposite side.

KNEELING RUNNERS POSE: Kneel on the floor. One leg with bent knee 90 degrees with foot on the ground. Other leg bent knee 90 degrees with shin laid flat on ground. Hands on hip push pelvic forward gently. Hold for 10-30 seconds. Repeat on opposite leg.

NECK / TRAP STRETCH: Sit on the floor in a cross-legged position or in a chair with feet flat on the ground.

Place hand on the top of your head and slowly tilt head to shoulder gently pulling head with hand. Apply gentle pressure with hand to increase and deepen the stretch.

Hold for 10-30 seconds, then slowly lift your head up and repeat stretch on the other side.

PECTORAL STRETCH: Standing tall with one forearm against a wall and elbow bent to 90 degrees. Gently turn your body away from the wall until a mild to moderate stretch is felt across chest. Hold for 10-30 seconds and repeat on the other side.

QUADRICEP STRETCH: Standing tall: back straight, shoulders back, facing forward. Use a chair or wall as needed for balance. Feet should be parallel and hip-width apart. Reaching back, grab one foot towards your buttocks, keeping your thighs aligned next to each other and opposite leg in line with your hip. Hold stretch for 10-30 seconds. Remember to breathe. Repeat with opposite leg.

SCIATIC STRETCH: 2 STRETCHES

1. Lie on your back with both legs extended on the ground. Keep both hips leveled so that your lower back is pressed down on the floor. Bend one knee, placing foot flat on the floor. Cross the opposite leg over the knee placing the ankle of extended leg above the bent knee. Grab the back of the thigh of the bent leg and gently hug towards chest. Breathe deeply and hold for 10-30 seconds. Repeat on opposite side.

2. **2.** Lie on your back with both legs extended on the ground. Keep both hips leveled so that your lower back is pressed down on the floor. Bend one knee towards your chest, grabbing it with opposite hand. Place your other hand out to the side. Keeping your shoulder blades squared on the floor use the opposite hand to guide the bent knee across body and towards the floor on opposite side. Hold

stretch for 10-30 seconds. Remember to breathe. Repeat with opposite leg.

SEATED SPINAL TWIST STRETCH: Sit on the floor with your legs straight out in front of you, glutes supported on a folded blanket/towel as needed. Bend knees, placing feet on the floor, then slide your right foot under your left leg to the outside of your left hip. Lay the outside of the right leg on the floor. Step the left foot over the right leg and stand it on the floor outside your right hip. The left knee will point directly up at the ceiling.

Exhale and twist toward the inside of the left thigh. Press the left hand against the floor just behind your left glute, and set your right upper arm on the outside of your left thigh near the knee. Pull your front torso and inner left thigh together.

Press the inner left foot very actively into the floor, release the left groin, and lengthen the front torso. Lean the upper torso back slightly, against the shoulder blades, and continue to lengthen the tailbone to the floor.

You can turn your head in one of two directions: Continue the twist of the torso by turning it to the left; or counter the twist of the torso by turning it right and looking over the right shoulder at the left foot. Hold stretch for 10-30 seconds then repeat on opposite side.

TRICEP STRETCH: Sit on a chair or stand with your back straight.

Raise your right arm straight overhead, and then bend it so your right hand is on the middle of your upper back. Your biceps and forearm should be touching.

Reach over with your left hand and grasp your right elbow on the top, so your left palm faces down.

Pull your right elbow gently toward your left side until you feel a stretch in your right triceps. Hold the stretch for 10 seconds and repeat on the other side.

Speak Life

Anger

I will refrain from anger and turn from wrath; I will not fret—it leads only to evil. (Psalm 37:8)

I will not take revenge, … but leave room for God's wrath, for it is written: "It is mine to avenge; I will repay," says the Lord. On the contrary: "If your enemy is hungry, feed him; if he is thirsty, give him something to drink. In doing this, you will heap burning coals on his head." I will not be overcome by evil, but evil with good. (Romans 12:19-21)

Comfort

The Lord is my refuge, a stronghold in times of trouble. (Psalm 9:9)

The Lord is my rock, my fortress and my deliverer. God is my rock that I take refuge in. He is my shield and the horn of my salvation, my stronghold. (Psalm 18:2)

I will wait for the Lord. I will be strong and take heart and wait for Him (Psalm 27:14)

Though I may stumble, I will not fall, for the Lord upholds me with His hand. (Psalm 37:24)

God is my refuge and strength, an ever-present help in trouble. Therefore I will not fear. (Psalm 46:1-3)

I cast my cares on the Lord; He sustains me and will never let me fall. (Psalm 55:22)

Though I walk in the midst of trouble, God preserves my life; He stretches out His hand against the anger of my enemies, and with His right hand, He saves me. (Psalm 138:7)

God will give me rest. (Matthew 11:28)

Through Christ, my comfort overflows. (2 Corinthians 1:5)

Contentment

My heart is at peace; it gives life to my body. (Proverbs 14:30)

I will not let my heart envy sinners I will always be zealous for the fear of the lord. There is surely a future hope for me, and my hope will not be cut off. (Proverbs 23:17-18)

I will keep my life free from the love of money and be content with what I have, because God said He would never leave me or forsake me.
(Hebrews 13:5)

Courage

I will wait for the Lord; I will be strong and take heart while I wait for the Lord. (Psalm 27:14)

I will be strong and courageous. I will not be terrified; I will not be discouraged for the Lord my God will be with me wherever I may go. (Joshua 1:9)

I will not fear for God has redeemed me, and has summoned me by name, I am His. (Isaiah 43:1)

Death/Loss

Even though I walk through the valley of the shadow of death, I will fear no evil, for you are with me; your rod and your staff, they comfort me.
(Psalm 23:4)

My flesh and my heart may fail, but God is the strength of my heart and my portion forever. (Psalm73:26)

For I am convinced that neither death nor life, neither angels nor demons, neither the present nor the future, nor any powers, neither height nor depth, nor anything else in all creation, will be able to separate me from the love of God that is in Christ Jesus my Lord. (Romans 8:38-39)

Enemies

For the Lord my God is the one who goes with me to fight for me against my enemies to give me victory. (Deuteronomy 20:4)

The Lord will grant that the enemies who rise up against me will be defeated before me. They will come at me in one direction but flee from me in seven. (Deuteronomy 28:7)

For in the day of trouble He will keep me safe in His dwelling; He will hide me in the shelter of His tabernacle and set me high upon a rock. Then my head will be exalted above the enemies who surround me; at his tabernacle I will sacrifice with shouts of joy; I will sing and make music to the Lord. (Psalm 27:5-6)

With God I will gain victory, and He will trample down my enemies.
(Psalm 60:12)

The Lord is with me; He is my helper. I will look in triumph on my enemies. (Psalm 118:7)

So I say with confidence, "The Lord is my helper; I will not be afraid. What can man do to me?" (Hebrews 13:6)

Faith

I live by faith, not by sight. (2 Corinthians 5:7)

I have been crucified with Christ and I no longer live, but Christ lives in me. The life I live in the body, I live by faith in the Son of God, who loved me and gave himself for me. (Galatians 2:20)

But the fruit of the Spirit is love, joy, peace, kindness, goodness, faithfulness, gentleness, and self-control. (Galatians 5:22-23)

...so that Christ may dwell in my heart through faith. I pray that I may be rooted and established in love, I may have power, together with the saints, to grasp how wide and long and high and deep is the love of Christ, and to know this love that surpasses knowledge—that I may be filled to the measure of all the fullness of God. (Ephesians 3:17-19)

Now faith is being sure of what we hope for and certain of what we do not see. (Hebrews 11:1)

Fear

Even though I walk through the valley of the shadow of death, I will fear no evil, for you are with me; your rod and your staff, they comfort me. You prepare a table before me in the presence of my enemies. You anoint my head with oil; my cup runs over. (Psalm 23:4-5)

The Lord is my light and my salvation—whom shall I fear? The Lord is my stronghold of my life—of whom shall I be afraid? Though an army besiege me, my heart will not fear; though war break out against me, even then will I be confident. (Psalm 27:1-3)

God is my refuge and strength, an ever-present help in trouble. (Psalm 46:1)

He will cover me with His feathers, and under His wings I will find refuge; His faithfulness will be my shield and rampart. I will not fear the terror of the night, nor the arrow that flies by day, nor the pestilence that stalks in the darkness, nor the plague that destroys at midday. (Psalm 91:4-6)

When I pass through the waters, God will be with me; and when I pass through the rivers, they will not sweep over me. When I walk through the fire, I will not be burned; the flames will not se me on fire. (Isaiah 43:2)

For God did not give me a spirit of fear, but a spirit of power, of love and of self-discipline. (2 Timothy 1:7)

No, in all these things I am more than a conqueror through Him who loved me. For I am convinced that neither death nor life, neither angels nor demons, neither the present nor the future, nor any powers, neither height nor depth, nor anything else in all creation, will be able to separate me from the love of God that is in Christ Jesus my Lord. (Romans 8:37-39)

So I say with confidence, "The Lord is my helper, I will not be afraid. What can man do to me?" (Hebrews 13:6)

No, in all these things I am more than a conqueror through Him who loved me. For I am convinced that neither death nor life, neither angels nor demons, neither the present nor the future, nor any powers, neither height nor depth, nor anything else in all creation, will be able to separate me from the love of God that is in Christ Jesus my Lord. (Romans 8:37-39)

Forgiveness

Do not say, "I'll pay you back for this wrong!" Wait for the Lord, and he will deliver you. (Proverbs 20:22)

But I tell you: Love your enemies and pray for those who persecute you, that you may be sons of your Father in heaven. He causes his sun to rise on the evil and the good, and sends rain on the righteous and the unrighteous. (Matthew 5:44-45)

For if you forgive men when they sin against you, your heavenly Father will also forgive you. (Matthew 6:14)

"And when you stand praying, if you hold anything against anyone, forgive him or her, so that your Father in heaven may forgive you of your sins. (Mark 11:25)

But love your enemies, do good to them, and lend to them without expecting to get anything back. Then your reward will be great, and you will be sons of the Most High, because He is kind to the ungrateful and wicked. Be merciful, just as your Father is merciful. "Do not judge, and you will not be judged. Do not condemn, and you will not be condemned. Forgive and you will be forgiven. Give, and it will be given to you. A good measure, pressed down, shaken together and running over, will be poured into your lap. For with the measure you use, it will be measured to you." (Luke 6:35-38)

On the contrary: "If your enemy is hungry, feed him, if he is thirsty, give him something to drink." (Romans 12:20)

God's Protection

I am His beloved, I rest secure in Him, for He shields me all day long, and I and the one the Lord loves, I rest between His shoulders."
(Deuteronomy 33:12)

I will laugh at destruction and famine, and need not fear the beasts of the earth. (Job 5:22)

I will be secure, because there is hope; I will look about you and take rest in your safety. I will lie down with no one to make me afraid, and many will court my favor. (Job 11:18-19)

I will lie down and sleep in peace, for you alone, O Lord, make me dwell in safety. (Psalm 4:8)

I will have no fear of bad news; my heart is steadfast, I trust in the lord. (Psalm 112:7)

The Lord will keep me from all harm –He will watch over my life; the Lord will watch over my coming and going both now and forevermore.
(Psalm 121:7-8)

When I lie down, I will not be afraid; when I die down, my sleep will be sweet. (Proverbs 3:24)

Gossip

Do not go about spreading slander among your people. Do not do anything that endangers your neighbor's life. I am the Lord. (Leviticus 19:16)

Keep your tongue from evil and your lips from speaking lies. (Psalm 34:13)

Your tongue plots destruction; it is like a sharpened razor, you who practice deceit. (Psalm 52:2)

A perverse man stirs up dissension, and a gossip separates close friends. (Proverbs 16:28)

The words of a gossip are like choice morsels; they go down to a man's inmost parts. (Proverbs 18:8)

A gossip betrays a confidence; so avoid a man who talks too much. (Proverbs 20:19)

As a north wind brings rain, so a sly tongue brings angry looks. (Proverbs25:23)

Without wood a fire goes out; without gossip a quarrel dies down. As charcoal to embers and as wood to fire, so is quarrelsome man for kindling strife. (Proverbs 26:20-21)

Guidance

God will instruct me and teach me in the way I should go; He will counsel me and watch over me. (Psalm 32:8)

For this God is my God forever and ever, He will be my guide even to the end. (Psalm 48:14)

God is always with me; He holds me by my right hand. He guides me with His counsel, and afterward He will take me into glory. (Psalm 73:23-24)

In all my ways I will acknowledge Him, and He will make my path straight. (Proverbs 3:6)

My God instructs me and teaches me the right way. (Isaiah 28:26)

Whether I turn to the right or to the left, my ears will hear a voice behind me, saying, "This is the way; walk in it." (Isaiah 30:21)

Help

From six calamities God will rescue me; in seven no harm will befall on me. (Job 5:19)

The Lord is my rock, my fortress, my deliverer; my God is my rock, in whom I take refuge. He is my shield and the horn of my salvation, my stronghold. (Psalm 18:2)

You, O Lord, keep my lamp burning; my God turns my darkness into light. (Psalm 18:28)

For He has not despised or disdained the suffering of my afflictions; He has not hidden His face from me but has listened to my cry for help.
(Psalm 22:24)

You are my hiding place; you will protect me from trouble and surround me with songs of deliverance. (Psalm 32:7)

Though I may stumble, I will not fall, for the Lord upholds me with His hand. (Psalm 37:24)

The salvation of the righteous comes from the Lord; He is my stronghold in time of trouble. (Psalm 37:39)

The Lord hears the needy and does not despise His captive people.

(Psalm 69:33)

Though You have made me see troubles, many and bitter, You will restore my life again; from the depths of the earth You will again bring me up. (Psalm 71:20)

For He will deliver the needy who cry out, the afflicted who have no one to help. He will take pity on the weak and the needy and save the needy form death. (Psalm 72:12-13)

My flesh and my heart may fail, but God is the strength of my heart and my portion forever. (Psalm 73:26)

Then no harm will befall on me, no disaster will come near my tent. For He will command His angels concerning me to guard me in all my ways.
(Psalm 91:10-11)

But He lifted the needy out of their affliction and increased their families like flocks. (Psalm 107:41)

Though I walk in the midst of trouble, You preserve my life, You stretch out Your hand against the anger of my foes, with Your right hand You save me. (Psalm 138:7)

Do not gloat over me, my enemy! Though I have fallen, I will rise. Tough I sit in darkness, the Lord will be my light. Because I have sinned against Him, I will bear the Lord's wrath, until He pleads my case and establishes my right. He will bring me out into the light; I will see His righteousness. (Micah 7:8-9)

Hope

I will be strong and take heart, all of my hope is in the Lord. (Psalm 31:24)

Why are you downcast, O my soul? Why so disturbed within me? I will put my hope in God, for I will yet praise Him, my Savior and my God.
(Psalm 42:11)

For You have been my hope, O Sovereign Lord, my confidence since my youth. (Psalm 71:5)

When calamity comes, the wicked are brought down, but even in death the righteous have a refuge. (Proverbs 14:32)

The faith and love that spring from the hope that is stored up for you in heaven and that you have already heard about in the word of truth, the gospel. (Colossians 1:5)

...which is Christ in me, the hope of glory. (Colossians 1:27)

Praise be to God and Father of our Lord Jesus Christ! In His great mercy He has given me a new birth into a living hope through the resurrection of Jesus Christ from the dead. (1 Peter 1:3)

Therefore, I will prepare my mind for action; be self-controlled; set my hope fully on the grace to be given to me when Jesus Christ is revealed.
(1 Peter 1:13)

Through Him I believe in God, who raised Him from the dead and glorified Him, and so my faith and my hope are in God. (1 Peter 1:21)

Everyone who has hope in Him purifies himself, just as He is pure. (1 John 3:3)

Joy

Surely then I will find delight in the Almighty and will lift up my face to God. (Job 22:26)

You have filled my heart with greater joy than when their grain and new wine abound. (Psalm 4:7)

In Him my heart rejoices, for I trust in His holy name. (Psalm 33:21)

My soul will be satisfied as with the richest of foods, with singing lips my mouth will praise You. (Psalm 63:5)

But I will rejoice in the Lord and glory in the Holy One of Israel.

(Isaiah 41:16)

I delight greatly in the Lord; my soul rejoices in my God. For He has clothed me with garments of salvation and arrayed me in a robe of righteousness, as a bridegroom adorns his head like a priest, and as a bride adorns herself with her jewels. (Isaiah 61:10)

Yet I will rejoice in the Lord, I will be joyful in God my Savior. (Habakkuk 3:18)

Loneliness

God is with me and will watch over me wherever I go. He will not leave me until He has done what He has promised me. (Genesis 28:15)

When I call on God, He will answer me, I will cry for help and He will say: Here am I. (Isaiah 58:9)

God will not leave me like an orphan. He will come to me. (John 14:18)

<u>Loving God</u>

I will delight myself in the Lord and He will give me my hearts desires. (Psalm 37:4)

"Because He loves me," says the Lord, "I will rescue him; I will protect him, for he acknowledges My name." (Psalm 91:14)

<u>Patience</u>

I will stand firm to the end and I will be saved. (Matthew 24:13)

Not only so, but I rejoice in my suffering, because I know that suffering produces perseverance; perseverance, character, and character, hope. (Romans 5:3-4)

I will not become weary in doing good, for at the proper time, I will reap a harvest if I do not give up. (Galatians 6:9)

May I hold unswervingly to the hope I profess, for He who promised is faithful. (Hebrews 10:23)

I need to persevere so that when I have done the will of God, I will receive what He has promised. (Hebrews10:36)

Consider it pure joy, my brothers, whenever you face trials of many kinds, because you know that the testing of your faith develops perseverance. Perseverance must finish its work so that you may be mature and complete, not lacking anything. (James 1:2-4)

…I too, will be patient and stand firm, because the Lord's coming is near. (James 5:7-8)

Peace

I will listen to what God the Lord will say; He promises peace to His people, His saints. (Psalm 85:8)

"Peace, peace, to those far and near," says the Lord. "And I will heal them." (Isaiah 57:19)

Peace I leave with you; My peace I give you. I do not give to you as the world gives. Do not let your hearts be troubled and do not be afraid.
(John 14:27)

I will let the peace of Christ rule in my heart, because I am a member of His one body, I am called to peace. And I will be thankful. (Colossians 3:15)

Now may the Lord of peace himself give me peace at all times and in every way. (2 Thessalonians 3:16)

Praise

Sing to the Lord! Give praise to the Lord! He rescues the life of the needy from the hands of the wicked. (Jeremiah 20:13)

Prayer

I will pray to God, and He will hear me. (Job 22:27)

When I call upon God in my day of trouble, He will deliver me and I will honor Him. (Psalm 50:15)

Evening, morning and noon I cry out in distress, and He hears my voice. (Psalm 55:17)

He will call upon me, and I will answer Him. (Psalm 91:15)

The Lord is near to me when I call on Him, He is near to all who call on Him in truth. He fulfills my desires because I fear Him; He hears my cry and saves me. (Psalm 145:18-19)

How gracious He will be when I cry for help! As soon as He hears, He will answer me. (Isaiah 30:19)

When I will call, and the Lord will answer; I will cry for help, and He will say: Here am I. (Isaiah 58:9)

Before I call God will answer, while I am still speaking He will hear.
(Isaiah 65:24)

Then when I call upon God, go to Him and pray to Him, He will listen to me. (Jeremiah 29:12)

When I call to God, He said He will answer and tell me great and unsearchable things I do not know. (Jeremiah 33:3)

When I ask and it will be given to me, if I seek I will find, when I knock He will open the door for me. For it is written that everyone who asks receives, those who seek finds; and those who knock, the door will be opened. (Matthew 7:7-8)

Whatever I ask for in prayer, and I believe, I will receive it, it will be mine. (Mark 11:24)

When I confess my sins and pray for others I will be healed because the prayer of a righteous man/woman is powerful and effective. (James 5:16)

I receive from Him anything I ask, because I obey His commands and do what pleases Him. (1 John 3:22)

This is the confidence I have in approaching God: that if I ask for anything according to His will, He hears me. And if I know that He hears me – whatever I ask – I know that I will have what I asked of Him.
(1 John 5:14-15)

Righteousness

From the Lord comes deliverance. May His blessings be on me. (Psalm 3:8)

Surely goodness and love will follow me all the days of my life, and I will dwell in the house of the Lord forever. (Psalm 23:6)

For the Lord God is my sun and shield; the Lord bestows favor and honor; no good thing does He withhold from me. (Psalm 84:11)

Seek God

The Lord is with me when I am with Him. If I seek Him, I will find Him… (2 Chronicles 15:2)

The gracious hand of God is on me when I look to Him… (Ezra 8:22)

The Lord is good to me because my hope is in Him also when I seek Him. (Lamentations 3:25)

I will seek the Lord and live. (Amos 5:4)

Shame

I will not be put to shame when I obey all of God's commands. (Psalm 119:6)

May my heart be blameless towards Your decrees, that I may not be put to shame. (Psalm 119:80)

Though I am suffering, I will not be ashamed because I know God, whom I believe, guards what I have entrusted to Him for today. (2 Timothy 1:12)

Though I suffer as a Christian, I am not ashamed but rather I will praise God because I bear His name. (1 Peter 4:16)

Trust

God is my refuge and strength, an ever-present help when I am in trouble. I will not fear. (Psalm 46:1-2)

The Lord God is a sun and shield, He bestows favor and honor on me. (Psalm 84:11-12)

I trust in the Lord and I do not lean on my own understanding; in all of my ways I acknowledge Him and He makes my paths straight. (Proverbs 3:5-6)

Relevant Bible Verses by Topic

<u>Obedience</u>

Deuteronomy 6:18 -Do what is right and good in the Lord's sight, so that it may go well with you and you may go in and take over the good land that the Lord promised on oath to your forefathers.

Deuteronomy 30:15-16 - See, I set before you today life and prosperity, death and destruction. For I command you today to love the Lord your God, to walk in his ways, and to keep His commands, decrees and laws; then you will live and increase, and the Lord your God will bless you in the land you are entering to posses.

Job 36:11 - If they obey and serve Him, they will spend the rest of their days in prosperity and their years in contentment.

Psalm 106:3 - Blessed are those who maintain justice, who constantly do what is right.

Matthew 5:19 - Anyone who breaks one of the least of these commandments and teaches others to do the same will be called least in the kingdom of heaven, but whoever practices and teaches the commands will be called great in the kingdom of heaven.

Matthew 7:21 - "Not everyone who says to me 'Lord, Lord' will enter the kingdom of heaven, but only those who do the will of my Father who is in heaven."

Matthew 7:24-25 - Therefore everyone who hears these words of mine and puts them into practice is like a wise man who built his house on the rock. The rain came down, the streams rose, and the winds blew and beat against that house; yet it did not fall, because it had its foundation on the rock."

John 5:24 - "I tell you the truth, whoever hears my word and believes Him who sent me has eternal life and will not be condemned; he has crossed over from death to life."

John 8:51 - "I tell you the truth, if anyone keeps my word, he will never see death."

Romans 8:28 - And we know that in all things God works for the good of those who love Him, who have been called according to His purpose.

Philippians 4:9 - Whatever you have learned or received or heard from me, or seen in me—put it into practice. And the God of peace will be with you.

1 John 2:17 - The world and its desires pass away, but the man who does the will of God lives forever.

1 John 3:22 - And receive from Him anything we ask, because we obey His commands and do what pleases Him.

Also see: Deuteronomy 5:29, 6:3, 7:12, 29:9, Hebrews 5:9, James 1:25, John 13:17, 15:10, Matthew 12:50, Romans 2:13

Power of the Word

Psalm 19:14 - Let the words of my mouth and the meditation of my heart be acceptable in your sight, O Lord, my rock and my redeemer.

Proverbs 12:18 – There is one whose rash words are lie sword thrusts, but the tongue of the wise brings healing.

Proverbs 13:3 – Whoever guards his mouth preserves his life; he who opens wide his lips come to ruin.

Proverbs 15:1 A soft answer turns away wrath, but a harsh word stirs up anger.

Proverbs 15:4 – A gentle tongue is a tree of life, but perverseness in it breaks the spirit.

Proverbs 18:21 – Death and life are in the power of the tongue, and those who LOVE it will eat its fruits.

Proverbs 21:23 – Whoever keeps his mouth and his tongue keeps himself out of trouble.

Matthew 12:36-37 – Tell you, on the day of judgment people will give account for every careless word they speak. For by your words you will be justified, and by your words you will be condemned.

Matthew 15:18 - But what comes out of the mouth proceeds from the heart, and this defiles a person.

Romans 12:14 – Bless those who persecute you, bless and do not curse them.

Ephesians 4:29 – Let no corrupting talk come out of your mouths, but only such as is good for building up, as fits the occasion, that it may give grace to those who hear.

Colossian 3:8 – But now you must put them all away: anger, wrath, malice, slander, and obscene talk from your mouth.

Also see: Colossians 4:6, Exodus 20:1-26, Genesis 15:1-21, James 1:26, 3:1-12, John 1:1, 1:14, Proverbs 15:2, 17:27-28, 25:11, 29:20

<u>Prayer</u>

Psalms 4:1 - Answer me when I call to you, O my righteous God. Give me relief from my distress; be merciful to me and hear my prayer.

Psalms 5:3 - In the morning, O LORD, you hear my voice; in the morning I lay my requests before you and wait in expectation.

Psalms 17:1- Hear, O LORD, my righteous plea; listen to my cry. Give ear to my prayer-- it does not rise from deceitful lips.

Psalms 37:7 -Be still before the LORD and wait patiently for him; do not fret when men succeed in their ways, when they carry out their wicked schemes.

Psalms 55:17 -Evening, morning and noon I cry out in distress, and he hears my voice.

Psalms 65:1-2 Praise awaits you, O God, in Zion; to you our vows will be fulfilled. O you who hear prayer, to you all men will come.

Psalms 145:18 - The LORD is near to all who call on him, to all who call on him in truth.

Proverbs 15:29 - The LORD is far from the wicked but he hears the prayer of the righteous.

Isaiah 55:6 - Seek the LORD while he may be found; call on him while he is near.

Matthew 5:43-44 - You have heard that it was said, 'Love your neighbor and hate your enemy.' But I tell you: Love your enemies and pray for those who persecute you

Matthew 7:7-8 - Ask and it will be given to you; seek and you will find; knock and the door will be opened to you. For everyone who asks receives; he who seeks finds; and to him who knocks, the door will be opened.

Matthew 7:11 - If you, then, though you are evil, know how to give good gifts to your children, how much more will your Father in heaven give good gifts to those who ask him!

Mark 11:24-25 - Therefore I tell you, whatever you ask for in prayer, believe that you have received it, and it will be yours. And when you stand praying, if you hold anything against anyone, forgive him, so that your Father in heaven may forgive you your sins."

John 14:13-14 - And I will do whatever you ask in my name, so that the Son may bring glory to the Father. You may ask me for anything in my name, and I will do it.

1 Corinthians 14:15 - So what shall I do? I will pray with my spirit, but I will also pray with my mind; I will sing with my spirit, but I will also sing with my mind.

Philippians 4:6 - Do not be anxious about anything, but in everything, by prayer and petition, with thanksgiving, present your requests to God.

Colossians 4:2 - Devote yourselves to prayer, being watchful and thankful.

1 Thessalonians 5:16-18 -Be joyful always; pray continually; give thanks in all circumstances, for this is God's will for you in Christ Jesus.

1 Timothy 2:8 - I want men everywhere to lift up holy hands in prayer, without anger or disputing.

Hebrews 4:16 - Let us then approach the throne of grace with confidence, so that we may receive mercy and find grace to help us in our time of need.

James 5:13-16 - Is any one of you in trouble? He should pray. Is anyone happy? Let him sing songs of praise. Is any one of you sick? He should call the elders of the church to pray over him and anoint him with oil in the name of the Lord. And the prayer offered in faith will make the sick person well; the Lord will raise him up. If he has sinned, he will be forgiven. Therefore confess your sins to each other and pray for each other so that you may be healed. The prayer of a righteous man is powerful and effective.

1 John 5:14-15 -This is the confidence we have in approaching God: that if we ask anything according to his will, he hears us. And if we know that he hears us--whatever we ask--we know that we have what we asked of him.

Also see: Ephesians 6:18-19, James 4:3, Luke 6:12, 11:1-4, 18:1-9, 1 Mark 11:17. 22-23, Matthew 6:5-12, Peter 3:7, Proverbs 15:8, 1Timothy 2:14, Revelation 5:8

Pride

Psalm 119:2 - You rebuke the arrogant, who are cursed and who stray from your commands.

Proverbs 8:13 - To fear the Lord is to hate evil; I hate pride and arrogance, evil behavior and perverse speech.

Proverbs 16:18 - Pride goes before destruction, a haughty spirit before a fall.

Proverbs 21:24 - Haughty eyes and a proud heart, the lamp of the wicked are sin!

Proverbs 26:12 - Do you see a man wise in his own eyes? There is more hope for a fool than for him.

Proverbs 27:2 - Let another praise you, and not your own mouth; someone else, and not your own lips.

Proverbs 28:25-26 - A greedy man stirs up dissension, but he who trusts in the Lord will prosper. He who trusts in himself is a fool, but he who walks in wisdom is kept safe.

Isaiah 5:21 - Woe to those who are wise in their own eyes and clever in their own sight.

Mark 9:35 - Sitting down, Jesus called the Twelve and said, "If any one wants to be first, he must be the very last, and the servant of all."

Luke 16:15 - He said to them, "You are the ones who justify yourselves in the eyes of men, but God knows your hearts. What is highly valued among men is detestable in God's sight."

John 5:44 - How can you believe if you accept praise from one another, yet make no effort to obtain the praise that comes from the only God?

2 Corinthians 10:17-18 - But, Let him who boasts boast in the Lord. For it is not the one who commends himself who is approved, but the one whom the Lord commends.

Also see: Job 40:12

<u>Repentance</u>

Psalm 34:18 – The Lord is close to the brokenhearted and saves those who are crushed in spirit.

Psalm 147:3 – He heals the brokenhearted and binds up their wounds.

Job 11:14-15 – If you put away that sin that is in your hand and allow no evil to dwell in your tent, then you will lift up your face without shame; you will stand firm and without fear.

Ezekiel 18:21-211 – "But if a wicked man turns away from all the sin he has committed and keeps all my decrees and does what is just and right, he will surely live; he will not die. None of the offenses he has committed will be remembered against him. Because of the righteous things he has done, he will live."

Mark 1:15 - "The time has come," he said. "The kingdom of God is near. Repent and believe the good news!"

Mark 6:12 – They went out and preached that people should repent.

<u>Self-Denial</u>

Matthew 5:39-41 – But I tell you, Do not resist an evil person. If someone strikes you on the right cheek; turn to him the other also. And if someone wants to sue you and take your tunic, let him have your cloak as well. If someone forces you to go one mile, go with him two miles.

Matthew 16:24-26 – Then Jesus said to his disciples, "If anyone would come after me, he must deny himself and take up his cross and follow me. For whoever wants to save his life will lose it, but whoever loses his life for me will find it. What good will it be for a man if he gains the whole world, yet forfeits his soul? Or what can a man give in exchange for his soul?"

Luke 18:29-30 – "I tell you the truth," Jesus said to them, "no one who has left home or wife or bothers or parents or children for the sake of the kingdom of God will fail to receive many times as much in this age and, in the age to come, eternal life."

Romans 8:12-13 - Therefore, brothers, we have an obligation – but it is not to the sinful nature, to live according to it, For if you live according to the sinful nature, you will die; but if by the Spirit you put to death the misdeeds of the body, you will live.

Galatians 5:24 – Those who belong to Christ Jesus have crucified the sinful nature with its passions and desires.

Titus 2:11-12 – For the grace of God that brings salvation has appeared to all men. It teaches us to say "No" to ungodliness and worldly passions, and to live self-controlled, upright, and godly lives in this present age.

<u>Slander and Reproach</u>

Psalm 31:20 – In the shelter of Your presence You hide them from the intrigues of men; in Your dwelling You keep them safe from accusing tongues.

Psalm 37:6 - He will make your righteousness shine like the dawn, the justice of your cause like the noonday sun.

Psalm 57:3 – He sends from heaven and saves me, rebuking those who hotly pursue me; God sends his love and His faithfulness.

Job 5:21 – You will be protected from the lash of tongue, and need not fear when destruction comes.

Isaiah 57:7 – Hear me, you who know what is right, you people who have my law in your hearts: Do not fear the reproach of men or be terrified by their insults.

Matthew 5:12-12 – Blessed are you when people insult you, persecute you, and falsely say all kinds of evil against you because of me. Rejoice and be glad, because great is your reward in heave, for in the same way they persecuted the prophets who were before you.

Also see: 1 Peter 4:14

<u>Success</u>

Psalm 40:4 - Blessed is the man who makes the Lord his trust.

Psalm 125:1 - Those who trust in the Lord are like Mount Zion, which cannot be shaken but endures forever.

Psalm 128:2 - You will eat the fruit of your labor; blessings and prosperity will be yours.

Proverbs 8:18-19 – With Me are riches and honor, enduring wealth and prosperity. My fruit is better than fine gold; what I yield surpasses choice silver.

Proverbs 15:6 - The house of the righteous contains great treasure, but the income of the wicked brings them trouble.

Proverbs 22:4 – Humility and the fear of the Lord bring wealth and honor and life.

Job 22:28 - What you decide on will be done, and light will shine on your ways.

1 Peter 5:7 -Cast your anxiety on Him because He cares about you.

Also see: Deuteronomy 11:15, 28:2-6, 28:11-13, 30:9, Ecclesiastes 3:13, 5:19, Isaiah 30:23, 65:21-23, Job 22:24-25, Psalm112:3

Trust

Psalm 37:3-5 - Trust in the Lord and do good; dwell in the land and enjoy safe pasture. Delight yourself in the Lord and He will give you the desires of your heart. Commit your ways to the Lord; trust in Him and He will do this.

Psalm 40:4 – Blessed is the man who makes the Lord his trust.

Psalm 46:1-2 – God is our refuge and strength, an ever-present help in trouble. Therefore we will not fear, though the earth give way and the mountains fall into the heart of the sea.

Psalm 84:11-12 – For the Lord God is a sun and shield; the Lord bestows favor and honor; no good thing does He withhold from those whose walk is blameless. O Lord Almighty, blessed is the man who trusts in You.

Psalm 125:1 - Those who trust in the Lord are like Mount Zion, which cannot be shaken but endures forever.

Mark 6:31-32 - So do not worry, saying, 'What shall we eat?' or 'What shall we drink?' or 'What shall we wear?' For the pagans run after all these things, and your heavenly Father knows that you need them.

Luke 12:32 - Do not be afraid little flock, for your Father has been pleased to give you the kingdom.

1 Peter 5:7 - Cast all your anxiety on Him because He cares for you.

Wisdom

James 1:5 - If any of you lacks wisdom, he should ask God, who gives generously to all without finding fault, and it will be given to him.

Isaiah 2:3 - He will teach us his ways, so that we may walk in his paths.

Psalm 32:8 - I will instruct you and teach you in the way you should go; I will counsel you and watch over you.

Ecclesiastes 2:26 - To the man who pleases him, God gives wisdom, knowledge and happiness.

Proverbs 2:5-7 – Then you will understand the fear of the Lord and find the knowledge of God. For the Lord gives wisdom, and from his mouth come knowledge and understanding. He holds victory in store for the upright, he is a shield to those whose walk is blameless.

Psalm 51:6 – Surely you desire truth in the inner parts; you teach me wisdom in the inmost place.

1 John 5:20 We know also that the Son of God has come and has given us understanding, so that we may know Him who is true- even in his Son Jesus Christ. He is the true God and eternal life.

Psalm 16:7 - I will praise the Lord, who counsels me; even at night my heart instructs me.

2 Corinthians 4:6 - For God, who said, "Let light shine out of darkness," made His light shine in our hearts to give us the light of the knowledge of the glory of God in the face of Christ.

Proverbs 28:5 – Evil men do not understand justice, but those who seek the Lord understand it fully.

Song List

As you listen to the songs, listen to the words;
hear what God has to say to you.
Sing the songs out loud. Sing the songs
to God; they are like prayers.

ARTIST	SONG
Addison Road	Change In The Making
Addison Road	Fight Another Day
Addison Road	Hope Now
Avalon	Alive
Big Daddy Weave	Audience Of One
Brandon Heath	Love Never Fails
Brandon Heath	The Light In Me
Britt Nicole	Hanging On
Britt Nicole	Have Your Way
Britt Nicole	Still That Girl (WOMEN)
Britt Nicole	Walk On The Water
Carrie Underwood	Jesus Take The Wheel
Carrie Underwood	Just Stand Up
Carrie Underwood	Lessons Learned
Carrie Underwood	Something In The Water
Carrie Underwood	So Small
Casting Crowns	Courageous (MEN)
Charlie Hall	Micah 6:8

Chris Tomlin	I Will Follow
Chris Tomlin	Unfailing Love
Chris Young	The Man I Want To Be (MEN)
Christina Aguilera	Beautiful
Chuck Prophet	No Other Love
David Crowder Band	Oh The Glory Of It All
David Guetta (feat Sia)	Titanium
Debra Captain	Hope
Debra Captain	Psalm 103
Destiny's Child	Survivor
Fee	Everything Falls
Fellowship Creative	Beautiful
Fireflight	For Those Who Wait
Florence & The Machine	Shake It Out
For King and Country	Busted Heart
Francesca Battistelli	He Knows My Name
Future Of Forestry	Close Your Eyes
Future Of Forestry	Protection
Future Of Forestry	Slow Your Breath
Gary Allan	Life Ain't Always Beautiful
Heather Williams	God Is Still Good
Hillsong United	Oceans
Jason Gray	Nothing Is Wasted
Jeremy Camp	He Knows
Jeremy Camp	I Still Believe
Jeremy Camp	There Will Be A Day
Jesse Blaze Snider	Go With Me (MEN)
Jessie J	Who You Are
Jonathan Clay	Heart On Fire
John Mayer	Say
John Waller	While I'm Waiting
Josh Wilson	Before The Morning
Josh Wilson	Savior, Please

Kari Jobe	Steady My Heart
Katy Perry	Roar
Kelly Clarkson	Stronger
Kenny Chesney	Some People Change
Kim Walker-Smith	Healing Oil
KT Tunstall	Suddenly I See
Kutless	Sea Of Faces
Kutless	What Faith Can Do
Lady Antebellum	I Was Here
Lecrae	God Is Enough
Lecrae	Rebel
Lecrae	Walk On Water
Lee Ann Womack	I Hope You Dance
Lifehouse	Everything
Love and The Outcome	He Is With Us
Mandisa	Overcomer
Martina McBride	Blessed
Matt Hammitt	All Of Me
Matt Maher	Lord I Need You
Matt Redman	10,000 Reasons
Matthew West	All The Broken Pieces
Matthew West	Family Tree
Matthew West	Forgiveness
Matthew West	Strong Enough
Mercy Me	The Hurt & The Healer
Meredith Andrews	Can Anybody Hear Me
Miley Cyrus	The Climb
Natalie Grant	Held
Natalie Grant	Hurricane
Need To Breathe	More Time
New World Son	Learning To Be The Light
Nickelback	If Today Was Your Last Day
One Direction	What Makes You Beautiful

Passion Band	The Heart Of Worship
Phil Wickham	Divine Romance
Phillip Phillips	Home
Pink	Perfect
Pink	Try
Point Of Grace	How You Live
Rachel Platten	Fight Song
Rob Thomas	Little Wonders
Sammy Kershaw	She Don't Know She's Beautiful
Sanctus Real	Lead Me
Sanctus Real	Pray
Sanctus Real	Whatever You're Doing
Selena Gomez	Who Says
Shawn McDonald	Have You Ever Wanted?
Sidewalk Prophets	Help Me Find It
Sidewalk Prophets	Lay Down My Life
Sidewalk Prophets	Words I Would Say
Story Side: B	Be Still
Switchfoot	This Is Your Life
Tenth Avenue North	Healing Begins
Tenth Avenue North	You Are More
The Goo Goo Dolls	Better Days
The Pogues	Love You Til The End
The Script (feat. Will.I.Am)	Hall of Fame
Third Day	Call My Name
Third Day	Can't Take The Pain
Third Day	Cry Out To Jesus
Third Day	Love Heals Your Heart
Third Day	Offering
Third Day	Praise You In This Storm
Tim McGraw	Better Than I Used To Be
Tim McGraw	Live Like You Were Dying
Tim McGraw	Still

Toby Mac	Get Back Up
Toby Mac	Speak Life
Todd Agnew	In The Middle Of Me
Warren Barfield	Love Is Not A Fight
33 Miles	One Life To Love

Acknowledgements

Thank you to my friends and family, both old and new, far and near, whom have supported me and helped me through each moment of this trying time with your prayers, your finances, and your words of encouragement, your blessings and your Love. Thank you to those who were strangers but took the chance to get to know me and I am now able to call my friends. Thank you to those who made time for me and shared their talents and knowledge, with me and my girls giving us opportunities we would not otherwise have had. There are not enough words to describe the joy and the thankfulness that my heart overflows with for you. Thank you also to the following people who helped me through this chapter of my life and those who helped to get my book to publication (in alphabetical order): Alisha Baker (trained me for my first competition), Amy Minor (for helping me to step back into the world), Arshay Cooper, author of Suga Water (guidance and friendship), Brooke Valls (author picture), Curtis Romano (for all of my supplements I needed for training for my 1ˢᵗ body building competition) Crystal Wright (for everything and for loving me unconditionally all of my life) Darrian and Daykota Rieg (enduring all of it with me and being their when I needed a hug), Deanna Storer (everything and always), Dimitrious Rieg (for being you), Donald Rieg (giving me your blessing to write and publish this book), Elizabeth Johnson (teaching me how to look and feel pretty again), Elizabeth Riddle (prayer partner and unconditional love), Chaplain Jason Owen (teaching and telling me to be thankful for my struggles and pain), Jennifer Hughes (standing in the gap), Jeremy Riddle (always making sure the girls and I had enough), Nick Brandeth (editing), Normal to Destiny (shirts), Sandra Dejardins (editing), Scott Wheeler (love and support and for always reminding me that I was and am God's Warrior Princess),Tom Carmine (cover help), the many backers of this book's Kickstarter, and my publisher, West Bow Press. I humbly ask for forgiveness for anyone I may have forgotten, your graciousness has meant so much to me.

Notes

Chapter 1: Rejection

- *"If the world hates you, know that it hated me before it hated you."* John 15:18 NIV

http://biblehub.com/john/15-18.htm

- *"Even there Your hand will lead me, And Your right hand will lay hold of me."* Psalm 139: 10 NASB

http://biblehub.com/psalms/139-10.htm

- *"for two will become one flesh. So they are no longer two, but one flesh."* Mark 10:8 NIV

http://biblehub.com/matthew/19-6.htm

- *"If a man vows a vow to the Lord, or swears an oath to bind himself by a pledge, he shall not break his word. He shall do according to all that proceeds out of his mouth."* Numbers 30:2 ESV

http://biblehub.com/numbers/30-2.htm

- *"The righteous cries out, and the Lord hears them; He delivers them from all of their troubles. The Lord is close to the broken hearted and saves those who are crushed in spirit."* Psalm 34:17-18 NIV

http://biblehub.com/psalms/34-17.htm
http://biblehub.com/psalms/34-18.htm

- *"The Lord is close to the brokenhearted and saves those who are crushed in spirit."* Psalm 34:18 NLT

https://www.biblegateway.com/passage/?search=psalm+34%3A18&version=NLT

- *"Then they cried to Lord in their trouble, and He saved them from their distress. He sent forth His word and healed them; He rescued them from the grave."* Psalm 107:19-20 NIV

http://biblehub.com/psalms/107-19.htm
http://biblehub.com/psalms/107-20.htm

Chapter 2: Choose

- *"This day I call the heavens and the earth as witness against you that I have set before you life and death, blessings and curses. Now choose life..."* Deuteronomy 30:19 NIV

http://biblehub.com/deuteronomy/30-19.htm

- *"No temptation has overtaken you except what is common to man; but God is faithful, He will not allow you to be tempted beyond what you are able, but with the temptation, He will make a way, so that you can endure it."* 1 Corinthians 10:13 NIV http://biblehub.com/niv/1_corinthians/10-13.htm

- *"everyone who calls on the name of the Lord will be saved."* Romans 10:13 NIV

http://biblehub.com/romans/10-13.htm

- *"Blessed is the man who remains steadfast under trial, for when he has stood the test he will receive the crown of life, which God has promised to those who love him."* James 1:12 ESV

http://biblehub.com/james/1-12.htm

- *"No temptation has overtaken you except such as is common to man; but God is faithful, who will not allow you to be tempted beyond what you are able, but with the temptation will also make the way of escape, that you may be able to bear it."* 1 Corinthians 10:13 NASB

http://biblehub.com/1_corinthians/10-13.htm

- *"So then each one of us will give an account of himself to God."* Romans 14:12 NASB

http://biblehub.com/nasb/romans/14.htm

- *"One day the angels came to present themselves before the LORD, and Satan also came with them"* Job 1:6 NIV

http://biblehub.com/job/1-6.htm

- *"The LORD said to Satan, 'Very well, then, everything he has is in your hands, but on the man himself do not lay a finger.' Then Satan went out from the presence of the LORD.*" Job 1:12 NIV

http://biblehub.com/job/1-12.htm

- "*I have said these things to you, that in me you may have peace. In the world you will have tribulation. But take heart; I have overcome the world.*" John 16:33 ESV

http://biblehub.com/john/16-33.htm

- "*All things, work together for the good for those who love Him, and are called according to His purpose.*" Romans 8:28 NIV

http://biblehub.com/romans/8-28.htm

- "*Just as the Son of Man did not come to be served, but to serve, and to give his life as a ransom for many.*" Matthew 20:28 NLT

https://www.biblegateway.com/passage/?search=matthew+ 20%3A28&version=NLT

- "*Carefully guard your thoughts because they are the source of true life.*" Proverbs 4:23 CEV

https://www.biblegateway.com/passage/?search=Proverbs+ 4%3A23&version=CEV

Chapter 3: Prayer

- "*For you have been a stronghold to the poor, a stronghold to the needy in his distress, a shelter from the storm and a shade from the heat.*" Isaiah 25:4 ESV http://biblehub.com/isaiah/25-4.htm

- *"Pour out your heart like water before the presence of the Lord!"* Lamentations 2:19 ESV

https://www.biblegateway.com/passage/?search=lamentations%20 2:19&version=ESV

- *"In my distress I called to the LORD; I cried to my God for help. From his temple he heard my voice; my cry came before him, into his ears."* Psalms 18:6

http://biblehub.com/psalms/18-6.htm

- *"be angry but do not sin."* Ephesians 4:26 ESV

http://biblehub.com/ephesians/4-26.htm

- *"I will take revenge; I will pay them back. In due time their feet will slip. Their day of disaster will arrive, and their destiny will overtake them."* Deuteronomy 32:35 NLT

http://biblehub.com/deuteronomy/32-35.htm

- *"Vengeance is mine, I will repay, says the Lord."* Romans 12:19 ESV

http://biblehub.com/romans/12-19.htm

- *"And will not God bring about justice for his chosen ones, who cry out to him day and night? Will he keep putting them off?"* Luke 18:7 NIV

https://www.biblegateway.com/passage/?search=luke+ 18%3A7&version=NIV

- *"You prepare a table before me in the presence of my enemies. You anoint my head with oil; my cup overflow."* Psalm 23:5 NIV

http://biblehub.com/psalms/23-5.htm

- *"Do not be deceived: God cannot be mocked. A man reaps what he sows."* Galatians 6:7 NIV

http://biblehub.com/galatians/6-7.htm

- *"One day the angels came to present themselves before the LORD, and Satan also came with them."* Job 1:6 NIV

http://biblehub.com/job/1-6.htm

- *"The LORD said to Satan, "Very well, then, everything he has is in your power, but on the man himself do not lay a finger." Then Satan went out from the presence of the LORD."* Job 1:12 NIV

http://biblehub.com/job/1-12.htm

- *"No temptation has overtaken you except what is common to mankind. And God is faithful; he will not allow you to be tempted beyond what you can bear. But when you are tempted, he will also provide a way out so that you can endure it."* 1 Corinthians 10:13 NIV

http://biblehub.com/1_corinthians/10-13.htm

- *"Be angry but do not sin."* Ephesians 4:26 ESV

http://biblehub.com/ephesians/4-26.htm

Chapter 4: Forgiveness

- *"Come out from among them and separate."* 2 Corinthians 6:17 MSG

https://www.biblegateway.com/passage/?search=2%20Corinthians+6%3A17

- *"Make allowances for each other's faults, and forgive anyone who offends you. Remember, the Lord forgave you, so you must forgive others."* Colossians 3:13 NLT

https://www.biblegateway.com/passage/?search=colossians+3%3A13&version=NLT

- *"Get rid of all bitterness, rage and anger, brawling and slander, along with every form of malice."* Ephesians 4:31 NIV

https://www.biblegateway.com/passage/?search=Ephesians+4%3A31&version=NIV

- *"Refrain from anger and turn from wrath; do not fret—it leads only to evil."* Psalm 37:8 NIV

http://biblehub.com/psalms/37-8.htm

- *"I will take revenge; I will pay them back. In due time their feet will slip. Their day of disaster will arrive, and their destiny will overtake them."* Deuteronomy 32:35 NLT

http://biblehub.com/deuteronomy/32-35.htm

- *"Beloved, never avenge yourselves, but leave it to the wrath of God, for it is written, "Vengeance is mine, I will repay, says the Lord."* Romans 12:19 ESV

http://biblehub.com/romans/12-19.htm

- *"Then the Master said, "Do you hear what that judge, corrupt as he is, is saying? So what makes you think God won't step in and work justice for his chosen people, who continue to cry out for help? Won't he stick up for them? I assure you, he will. He will not drag his feet. But how much of that kind of persistent faith will the Son of Man find on the earth when he returns?"* Luke 18:7 MSG

http://biblehub.com/parallel/luke/18-7.htm

- *"For the eyes of the LORD move to and fro throughout the earth that He may strongly support those whose heart is completely His..."* 2 Chronicles 16:9 NASB

https://www.biblegateway.com/passage/?search=2+chronicles+16%3A9&version=NASB

- *"I will take revenge; I will pay them back. In due time their feet will slip. Their day of disaster will arrive, and their destiny will overtake them."* Deuteronomy 32:35 NLT

https://www.biblegateway.com/passage/?search=2+chronicles+16%3A9&version=NASB

- *"Beloved, never avenge yourselves, but leave it to the wrath of God, for it is written, "Vengeance is mine, I will repay, says the Lord."* Romans 12:19 ESV https://www.biblegateway.com/passage/?search=romans+12%3A19&version=ESV

- *"Then the Master said, "Do you hear what that judge, corrupt as he is, is saying? So what makes you think God won't step in and work justice for his chosen people, who continue to cry out for help? Won't he stick up for them? I assure you, he will. He will not drag his feet. But how much of that kind of persistent faith will the Son of Man find on the earth when he returns?"* Luke 18:6-8 MSG

https://www.biblegateway.com/passage/?search=luke+18%3A7&version=MSG

- *"You prepare a table before me in the presence of my enemies; you anoint my head with oil; my cup overflow."* Psalm 23:5 ESV

http://biblehub.com/psalms/23-5.htm

- *"Truthful words stand the test of time and lies will soon be exposed."* Proverbs 12:19 NLT

http://www.biblestudytools.com/nlt/proverbs/12-19.html

- *"There is nothing concealed that will not be disclosed, or hidden that will not be made known."* Luke 12:2 NIV

http://biblehub.com/luke/12-2.htm

- *"My God, my God, why have you forsaken me?"* Matthew 27:46 NIV

http://biblehub.com/matthew/27-46.htm

Chapter 5: Praise and Gratitude

- *"It is a good thing to give thanks unto the Lord, and to sing praises unto thy name, O Most High."* Psalm 92:1 KJV

http://biblehub.com/psalms/92-1.htm

- Psalm 145 KJV

http://biblehub.com/psalms/145-1.htm

Chapter 6: Trust

- *"Trust in the Lord with all your heart; and lean not on your own understanding. In all your ways acknowledge Him and He will make your paths straight."* Proverbs 3:5-6 AMP

http://biblehub.com/proverbs/3-5.htm
http://biblehub.com/proverbs/3-6.htm

- *"For the word of the Lord is right and true; he is faithful in all he does."* Psalm 33:4 NIV

http://biblehub.com/psalms/33-4.htm

Chapter 7: Action

- *"Set your mind on things above, not on earthly things."* Colossians 3:2 NIV

http://biblehub.com/colossians/3-2.htm

- *"…but I focus on this one thing: Forgetting the past and looking forward to what lies ahead,"* Philippians 3:13 NLT https://www.biblegateway.com/passage/?search=Philippians+3%3A13&version=NLT

- *"Think on things that are true, noble, right, pure, lovely, admirable, excellent or praise worthy."* Philippians 4:8 KJV

http://biblehub.com/philippians/4-8.htm

- *A good man/woman brings good things stored up in his/her heart, and an evil man/woman brings evil things stored up in his/her heart. For the mouth speaks what the heart is full of."* Luke 6:45 NIV

http://biblehub.com/luke/6-45.htm

- *"Each of you must take responsibility for doing the creative best you can with your own life."* Galatians 6:5 AMP

http://biblehub.com/galatians/6-5.htm

- *"Get rid of all bitterness, rage and anger, brawling and slander, along with every form of malice. Be kind and compassionate to one another, forgiving each other, just as in Christ God forgave you."* Ephesians 4:31-32 NIV

http://biblehub.com/ephesians/4-31.htm
http://biblehub.com/ephesians/4-32.htm

- *"The tongue has the power of life and death, and those who love it will eat its fruit."* Proverbs 18:21 NIV

http://biblehub.com/proverbs/18-21.htm

- *"Death and life are in the power of the tongue."* Proverbs 18:21 ESV http://biblehub.com/proverbs/18-21.htm

- *"The righteous must choose their friends carefully, for the way of the wicked leads them astray."* Proverbs 12:26 ESV

https://www.biblegateway.com/passage/?search=proverbs+12%3A26&version=ESV

- "If you "walk with wise men you become wise." Proverbs 13:20 NASB

http://bible.knowing-jesus.com/Proverbs/13/20

- *"Do not become friends with angry people or be associated with them or you will become like them."* Proverbs 22:24 NLT

http://biblehub.com/proverbs/22-24.htm

- *"Become wise by walking with the wise; hangout with fools and watch your life fall to pieces."* Proverbs 13:20 MSG

https://www.biblegateway.com/passage/?search=proverbs+13%3A20&version=MSG

- *"Therefore, be careful how you walk, not as an unwise man but as wise, making the most of your time…"* Ephesians 5:15-16 NASB

http://biblehub.com/ephesians/5-15.htm
http://biblehub.com/ephesians/5-16.htm

Chapter 8: Redemptive Love

- *All things do work together for the good to those who love God, to those who are called according to HIS purpose."* Romans 8:28 ESV

https://www.biblegateway.com/passage/?search=Romans%20 8:28&version=ESV

- *"Blessed is she who has believed that the Lord would fulfill His promises to her."* Luke 1:45 NIV

http://biblehub.com/luke/1-45.htm

- *"We love him because he first loved us."* 1 John 4:19 KJV

http://biblehub.com/1_john/4-19.htm

Chapter 9: Repentance

- *"Repent, then, and turn to God, so that your sins may be wiped out, that times of refreshing may come from the Lord"* Acts 3:19 NIV

http://biblehub.com/acts/3-19.htm

CPSIA information can be obtained
at www.ICGtesting.com
Printed in the USA
FSOW01n0752170217
30946FS